Praise for

AS NATURE MADE HIM

"An object lesson in medical hubris and close-the-ranks collusion, and in the tragic results when ideology trumps common sense in thinking about sex and gender. Above all, it's a deeply moving human drama and a testament to the inner strength and courage of the child who never lost touch with who he really was."

—DEBORAH TANNEN,
author of *You Just Don't Understand*

"Harrowing and enthralling. . . . Makes a convincing case that gender has less to do with the signals we send and receive from the world than with ineradicable messages encoded in every cell of our brains and bodies."

—*Elle*

AS
NATURE
MADE HIM

AS NATURE MADE HIM

≡

The Boy Who Was Raised as a Girl

JOHN COLAPINTO

Perennial

An Imprint of HarperCollins*Publishers*

Portions of this book were originally published in *Rolling Stone*.

A hardcover edition of this book was published in 2000 by HarperCollins Publishers.

First Perennial edition published 2001.

Designed by Elliott Beard

The Library of Congress has catalogued the hardcover edition as follows:

Colapinto, John.
    As nature made him : the boy who was raised as a girl/John Colapinto—1st ed.
      p. cm.
    ISBN 0-06-019211-9
    1. Transsexuals—Canada—Biography. 2. Sex change—Case studies. 3. Gender identity. 4. Nature and nurture. I. Title.
RC560.G45C65 2000
305.9'066 B—dc21   99-40167

ISBN 0-06-092959-6 (pbk.)

01 02 03 04 05 ❖/RRD 10 9 8 7 6 5 4 3 2 1

To Donna

I have entered on an enterprise which is without precedent, and will have no imitator. I propose to show my fellows a man as nature made him, and this man shall be myself.

—ROUSSEAU, *Confessions*

How could I not be glad to know my birth?

—SOPHOCLES, *Oedipus Rex*

The difficulty is to detach the framework of fact—of absolute undeniable fact—from the embellishments of theorists and reporters. Then, having established ourselves upon this sound basis, it is our duty to see what inferences may be drawn and what are the special points upon which the whole mystery turns.

—*Memoirs of Sherlock Holmes*

Author's Note

=

THIS IS A WORK OF NONFICTION. All passages of dialogue are taken verbatim from tape transcripts of psychological interviews, from contemporaneous psychiatric session notes, or from the direct recollection of witnesses to, or participants in, these events. No dialogue or scenes have been invented for the purposes of "narrative flow," "atmosphere," or any other quasi-novelistic purpose. The account of Dr. Money's appearance on the Canadian Broadcasting Corporation television show in 1967 is taken from a videotape of that program—a tape that was, miraculously, not destroyed in the thirty years since its broadcast. Direct dialogue from the Psychohormonal Research Unit sessions (published here for the first time) is taken from tape transcripts which Dr. Money supplied to the patient in June 1998 upon the request of the patient's local physician.

Preface

≡

On the morning of 27 June 1997 I paid my first visit to David Reimer's home, a small, nondescript dwelling in a working-class neighborhood of Winnipeg, Manitoba. There was nothing about the house to suggest that its owner might arouse the interest of a journalist from New York City—not to mention the fascination of scientists and doctors the world over. On the well-tended lawn, a child's bicycle lay on its side. At the curb was parked an eight-year-old secondhand Toyota. Inside the house, a handmade wooden cabinet in a corner of the living room held the standard emblems of family life: wedding photos and school portraits, china figurines, and souvenirs from family trips. There was a knock-off antique coffee table, a worn easy chair, and a sofa—which was where my host, a wiry young man dressed in a jean jacket and scuffed work boots, seated himself.

At thirty-one years of age David Reimer could have passed for more than a decade younger. Partly it was the sparseness of his facial hair—just a few blond wisps that sprouted from his jawline; partly it was a certain delicacy to his prominent cheek-bones and tapering chin. Otherwise he looked and sounded like what he was: a blue-collar factory worker, a man of high school education, whose fondest pleasures were to do a little weekend fishing with his dad in the local river or to have a backyard barbecue with his wife and kids. He was the kind of rough-edged but affable young man whose conversation ran to such topics as his tinkering with his car engine, his work woes, or the challenges of raising three kids on less than forty thousand a year.

I had come to Winnipeg to learn all I could about David Reimer, but my chief interest was in his childhood—a subject that, when I raised it, brought an immediate and dramatic change in him. Gone was the smile on his face and the bantering tone in his voice. Now his brows gathered together above his small straight nose, his eyes began to blink with startled rapidity, and he thrust his chin forward like someone who'd just been challenged to a fight. His voice—a deep, burred baritone—took on a new pitch and rhythm, an insistent, hammering rhythm, which for all its obvious aggrievement and anger also carried the pleading edge of someone desperate to communicate emotions that he feared others could never understand. How well even *he* understood these emotions was not immediately clear. I noticed that when David described events that had occurred prior to his fifteenth birthday, he tended to drop the pronoun *I* from his speech, replacing it with the distancing *you*—almost as if he were speaking about someone else altogether. Which, in a sense, he was.

"It was like brainwashing," he was saying as he lit the first in an unbroken chain of cigarettes. "I'd give just about anything to go to a hypnotist to black out my whole past. Because it's torture. What they did to you in the body is sometimes not near as bad as what they did to you in the *mind*—with the psychological warfare in your head."

He was referring to the events that had begun to unfold on an April morning three decades earlier when, at eight months of age, he lost his entire penis to a botched circumcision. As a result of that irreparable injury, his parents had taken him to see a famed expert in sex research at the renowned Johns Hopkins Hospital in Baltimore where they were convinced to submit their son to a surgical sex change. The process involved clinical castration and other genital surgery when he was a baby, followed by a twelve-year program of social, mental, and hormonal conditioning to make the transformation take hold in his psyche. The case was reported in the medical literature as an unqualified success, and he became one of the most famous (though unnamed) patients in the annals of modern medicine.

It was a fame that derived not only from the fact that his medical and surgical metamorphosis from boy to girl was the first infant sex reassignment ever reported on a developmentally normal child, but also from a stunning statistical long shot that lent special significance to the case. He had been born an identical twin. His brother and sole sibling provided to the experiment a built-in matched control—a genetic clone who, with penis and testicles intact, was raised as a male. That the twins were reported to have grown into happy, well-adjusted children of opposite sex seemed unassailable proof of the primacy of environment over biology in the differentiation of the sexes. Textbooks in medicine and the social sciences were rewritten to include the case, and a precedent for infant sex reassignment as standard treatment in cases of newborns with injured or irregular genitals was established. The case also became a touchstone for the feminist movement in the 1970s, when it was widely cited as proof that the gender gap was purely a result of cultural conditioning, not biology. For Dr.

John Money, the medical psychologist who was the architect of the experiment, the so-called "twins case" became the most publicly celebrated triumph of a forty-year career that in 1997 earned him the accolade "one of the greatest sex researchers of the century."

But as the mere existence of the young man who sat in front of me on that morning in June 1997 would suggest, the experiment was a failure—a fact not publicly revealed until that spring, in the medical journal *Archives of Pediatrics and Adolescent Medicine*. There, authors Dr. Milton Diamond, a biologist at the University of Hawaii, and Dr. Keith Sigmundson, a psychiatrist from Victoria, British Columbia, had documented how David had struggled against his imposed girlhood from the start and how, at age fourteen, he had reverted to the sex written in his genes and chromosomes. The paper had set off shock waves in medical circles around the world, generating furious debate about the ongoing practice of infant sex reassignment (a procedure more common than a layperson might think). The paper also raised troubling questions about the way the case had been reported in the first place, why it had taken almost twenty years for a follow-up to reveal the actual outcome, and why that follow-up was conducted not by Dr. Money or Johns Hopkins, but by outside researchers. The answers to these questions, fascinating for what they suggest about the mysteries of sexual identity, also brought to light a thirty-year rivalry between eminent sex researchers, a rivalry whose very bitterness not only dictated how this most unsettling of medical tragedies was exposed, but also may have been the impetus behind the experiment in the first place.

What was shaping up for medicine to be a highly public scandal involving some of the biggest names in the world of sex research was for David Reimer a purely private catastrophe.

Apart from two television interviews that he granted in the summer of 1997 (his face obscured, his voice disguised), he had never told his story in full to a journalist. He had agreed to speak to me, for an article I was preparing on the case for *Rolling Stone* magazine, on the condition that I withhold crucial details of his identity. Accordingly, in the article I did not reveal where he was born, raised, and continued to live, and I invented pseudonyms for his parents, Ron and Janet, and for his identical twin brother, Brian. The physicians who treated him in Winnipeg, I identified by initials. David himself I called, variously, "John" and "Joan," the pseudonyms given to him by Diamond and Sigmundson in their journal article describing the macabre double life he had been obliged to lead. So careful was I to provide not even the most oblique clue to David's geographic whereabouts that I omitted even to mention the historic blizzard that paralyzed Winnipeg on the morning of his circumcision accident—a freak late April snowfall eerily evocative of those reversed natural wonders that always presage horror in Shakespearean and Greek tragedies.

My *Rolling Stone* article appeared in December 1997. At nearly twenty thousand words, it was as thorough a job as could be managed under the space constraints and deadline pressures of magazine journalism. But even as the piece went to press, it was clear that David's life and the scientific machinations that played such a decisive part in shaping it were of sufficient complexity, scientific import, and human drama to require, for their fullest telling, a book. David, it transpired, had been thinking along the same lines and wanted me to be the book's author. At which point I was obliged to reveal to him an important condition for my taking on the project: that he abandon the mask of John/Joan.

Quite apart from the fact that I could not imagine writing a book in which the central character, his family, friends, physi-

cians, and others exist as pseudonyms moving against the inde-
terminate background of a "city somewhere in the North
American Midwest," I also knew that a knowlege of his specific
geographic location and the people who inhabited it were considered vital to a proper understanding of the case. In a tale at
the very heart of which lies the debate surrounding nature versus nurture, genetics versus environment, biology versus rearing, it was imperative that I be permitted to describe in detail
the sociocultural milieu in which David was raised. Finally, as a
writer, I knew how many of the story's peculiarly poetic reso-
nances would be lost should David insist upon anonymity. To
stick to pseudonyms would mean forfeiting the story of how
David, when beginning his laborious switch back to boyhood
at age fourteen, had rechristened himself with a male name different from his original birth name of Bruce—one that not only
had the kind of down-to-earth masculine directness he favored,
but also evoked for him his accomplishment in triumphing over
the array of forces that had conspired, for the first fourteen
years of his life, to convince him that he was someone other
than the person he felt himself inwardly to be. It was owing to
this unlikely victory that he had decided to name himself after
the child in the Bible story who slew the seemingly invincible
giant Goliath. Here, and in myriad other instances, to retain
pseudonyms was to sacrifice a fact that reflected not only on the
saga as a whole, but on David's own understanding of it.

Beginning with the interviews he had first granted to Diamond and Sigmundson in early 1993 for their journal article
and continuing with the interviews he gave to me for *Rolling
Stone*, David had been moving by degrees out of the shadows
of shame and secrecy in which he had been living. By the time I
spoke to him about abandoning the mask of John/Joan, he had
already come a long way in that journey. After discussing it
with his wife, parents, and brother, and sleeping on it for one

night, David told me that he was ready to step forward as his true self.

For the purposes of my reconstructing his past, David closed no doors, shut down no avenue of inquiry. He granted me over one hundred hours of interviews spread over twelve months, and he signed confidentiality waivers giving me access to an array of private legal papers, therapy notes, Child Guidance Clinic reports, IQ tests, medical records, and psychological workups that had accumulated over the course of his remarkable childhood. He assisted me in finding the schoolteachers and classmates who had known him in childhood—a difficult task of sleuthing since he had kept no school yearbooks, remembered few of his peers' last names, and had spent the previous decade and a half trying to forget and avoid anyone who had known him in his previous incarnation as a girl. Most crucially, David helped me obtain interviews with all of his family members, including his father, who because of the painfulness of these events had not spoken of them to anyone in more than twenty years. It is only through the Reimer family's rare candor that the full story of John/Joan can finally be told. Although that story is primarily about David Reimer and his experience of living on both sides of the gender divide, it is also about the young couple who, barely out of their teens, made the momentous decision to submit one of their twin baby boys to this unprecedented, and ultimately doomed, experiment in psychosexual engineering.

"My parents feel very guilty, as if the whole thing was their fault," David explained to me during my first visit to Winnipeg. "But it wasn't like that. They did what they did out of *kindness* and love and desperation. When you're desperate, you don't necessarily do all the right things."

PART ONE

A Game of Science Fiction

I

≡

The irony was that Ron and Janet Reimer's life together had begun with such special promise. That it would survive its trials is attributable perhaps in part to their shared heritage in an ethnic and religious background virtually defined by the hardiness of its people in the face of suffering.

Both Ron Reimer and Janet Schultz were descended from families who were Mennonite, the Anabaptist sect founded in sixteenth-century Holland. Like the Amish, Ron's and Janet's Mennonite ancestors were pacifists who followed a simple, nonworldly life based directly on Christ's teachings in the Sermon on the Mount. During the Inquisition, Mennonites were tortured and slaughtered in the thousands, the survivors escaping to begin a three-hundred-year search for a country that would allow them to live as a culture and religion apart. The majority went to Russia and farmed, but in the late 1800s, large numbers began to migrate to the New World, some settling in Nebraska and Kansas. The densest concentrations, however, settled in Canada, where the federal government, eager to populate its empty western plains, offered to the Mennonites complete religious freedom, their own schools, and exemption from military service. The first Mennonites arrived in southern Manitoba in 1874. Within five years, over ten thousand had followed, transplanting entire Russian villages to the Canadian prairie. It was in this wave of immigrants that both Ron's and Janet's great-grandparents, who were Dutch Mennonites directly descended from the earliest followers of the sect, came to Manitoba.

Their arrival coincided with that moment when the Canadian Pacific Railway reached Winnipeg, and transformed the once tiny and isolated fur-trapping settlement and Hudson's Bay trading post. Within three decades the settlement had become a major grain capital of the North American middle west. "All roads lead to Winnipeg," the *Chicago Record Herald* reported in 1911. "It is destined to become one of the greatest distributing commercial centers of the continent as well as a manufacturing community of great importance."

Though the city failed to live up to those grand predictions, Winnipeg did grow rapidly in size, sophistication, and importance over the first half of the twentieth century, establishing the country's first national ballet company and symphony orchestra. Today its population is over 600,000, and the city's downtown core, built around the meandering curves of the Red River, boasts an impressive stand of modern high-rises to complement its fine Victorian buildings.

The Mennonites on the surrounding prairies had long felt the lure of Winnipeg's affluence, and after World War II the more assimilated families began to move into the city to take jobs in manufacturing, trucking, and construction. Among them were Ron Reimer's parents, Peter and Helen, who in 1949 sold their farm in nearby Deloraine and moved to the Winnipeg neighborhood of St. Boniface, where Peter took a job in a slaughterhouse and Helen raised their four young children, of whom Ron was the eldest.

Even as a small child, he was dutiful and hardworking, a boy whose combination of personal privacy and dogged industry often amazed his own mother. "He was always so shy and quiet," Helen Reimer recalls, "but he was also such a *busy* little boy. I had to think up ways to keep him out of trouble. I would show him how to cook. He always wanted to be doing something with food and cooking." It was a passion that would stay with Ron. As an adult he would eventually support his wife and two children by running his own business as the operator of a coffee truck, supplying sandwiches and other prepared foods to construction sites around Winnipeg.

By 1957, when Ron was in his early teens, the music of Elvis Presley, Chuck Berry, and Little Richard had reached Winnipeg. Cars, girls, beer, and rock 'n' roll music soon had strong claims on his attention. For Mennonites of Ron's parents' generation, the swift cultural changes of the late 1950s were threatening. Though not themselves especially devout, they had only a decade earlier moved from an almost exclusively Mennonite farm community where some of the day-to-day values and assumptions were still closer to those of nineteenth-century rural Russia than late-twentieth-century urban North America. In what would prove to be a kind of reverse migration, the Reimers were among many Mennonite families who, in an effort to resist the seismic cultural shifts taking place in the city, returned their families to their roots on the prairie. In 1959, Ron's father bought a farm some sixty miles from the city, near the town of Kleefeld, in Mennonite country, and moved his family there.

Ron, fifteen years old at the time, hated the move. Kleefeld itself was little more than a ramshackle scattering of stores along a few hundred yards of gravel highway (grain store, post office, grocery), with nowhere for Ron to channel his formidable work ethic. He would pick two hundred pounds of saskatoons and sell them for twenty-five cents a pound—grueling labor for little pay; nothing like the money he was able to make in the city. And his father insisted on taking even those paltry sums from Ron for upkeep of the old clapboard farmhouse on its patch of scrubby land.

It was in this state of boredom, penury, and growing friction with his strict and authoritarian father that Ron, at seventeen, accepted the invitation of his friend Rudy Hildebrandt to visit Rudy's girlfriend in the nearby town of Steinbach. Rudy's girlfriend had a nice-looking roommate, a girl named Janet, whom Ron might like.

Like Ron, Janet Schultz was raised in Winnipeg, the eldest child of Mennonite parents who had joined the postwar migration from the prairie to the city. Growing up in the Winnipeg neighborhood of St. Vital, Janet was a lively and inquisitive girl whose passion for reading—first Nancy Drew and Hardy Boys books, then thrillers, and eventually books on psychology—opened up for her a perspective on life beyond the traditional Mennonite values of her parents—and in particular her mother, with whom she constantly clashed. "I wanted an education, but my mother wanted me to get out to work and bring home money," Janet says. Eventually she was convinced to quit school after ninth grade and take a job at a sewing factory. Janet gave her paychecks to her mother, which did little to foster goodwill between them. A further gulf opened between mother and daughter when Janet, in her early teens, stopped attending the Mennonite church. "I found it was so restrictive," she says. "I didn't think it was biblical. They said it was a sin to smile. I didn't think that way." In fact, by age fifteen, Janet was given to joking about her parents' religion. "Why don't Mennonites ever make love standing up?" she liked to ask her friends. "Because someone might think they were *dancing*!" Janet herself loved to go dancing and roller-skating, and as an exceptionally pretty hazel-eyed brunet with a shapely figure, she never lacked for dates.

Convinced that their eldest child and only daughter was slipping dangerously from their control, Janet's parents, like Ron Reimer's, joined the migration of city Mennonites back to the farm. In 1960, when Janet was fourteen, the Schultzes relocated to New Bothwell, a tiny settlement amid the silos and grain fields forty-five minutes from Winnipeg. Janet missed the city's movie theaters, restaurants, roller rinks, and dance halls—and soon began accepting dates from any boy who had a car and thus could offer her escape from the farm. Janet's mother tried to curb her daughter's social life but to no avail. Shortly after Janet's fifteenth birthday, her mother told her to move out. Janet went gladly. She moved to the nearby city of Steinbach, where she found work at a sewing factory and shared a small apartment in a rooming house with her cousin Tina. Not long after that, Tina's boyfriend brought a young man over to meet Janet. He was a tall blond boy of seventeen with large blue eyes and a shy way of glancing at her. His name was Ron Reimer. "I was flirting with Ron," she says, laughing, "and I was thinking he wasn't flirting back, so I figured he didn't like me."

Ron *did* like her, but was too shy to reveal his feelings in front of the other couple. He invited Janet to have a look at his car on the street, then asked her out to see a movie on the weekend. He raised money for their date by taking the transmission out of a junkyard Ford and selling it to a friend for ten dollars. That weekend, Ron and Janet went to see *Gidget Goes Hawaiian*. "I don't think I watched five minutes of that movie," Janet laughs. "I was too busy eyeballing him. Oh, he was so sexy!"

Over the course of the summer they saw a lot of each other,

joining Tina and Rudy on double dates—usually just a drive
out to one of the isolated country roads where they would park,
drink a six-pack, make out, and talk. As Ron and Janet compared their backgrounds, they were amazed to discover how
much they had in common. Their similarities drew them
together, but paradoxically enough so did their differences.
Janet could compensate for Ron's sometimes passive reluctance
to take decisive action; Ron, on the other hand, with his slow,
considered approach to life, could rein Janet in from her more
reckless enthusiasms and impulses. Together they made up a
single entity stronger than either one of them.

When Janet decided to move back into Winnipeg, there was
never any question but that Ron would follow her. Though
they did not rent an apartment together—this was the early
1960s, and such boldness would have been unthinkable for a
pair not yet out of their teens—Ron did spend much of his time
with Janet in her rooming house. It was there that they slept
together for the first time. Both had been virgins. And not long
after that, Janet missed her period. She had just turned eighteen. Ron was nineteen, soon to turn twenty. It was young to
marry, but they had talked about marriage before. This was
simply a sign that they should bless their union sooner rather
than later. The two were married on 19 December 1964 in the
city of Steinbach. In acknowledgment of the emancipation they
now felt from their disapproving parents, they deliberately
declined to be married in one of the city's twenty Mennonite
churches.

The newlyweds moved into a tiny cold-water flat in downtown Winnipeg. They couldn't afford better. Janet was getting minimum wage working as a waitress at the Red Top
diner; Ron was toiling for low pay at a factory that made
windows. That they would have to bring in more money was
obvious—especially when, during one of Janet's checkups

with her obstetrician, she learned that she was pregnant with twins. Ron was nervous, but Janet refused to be anything but optimistic. "I was so excited," she says, "because all my life I'd been dreaming, Oh wouldn't it be wonderful to have twins?"

That June, when Janet was five months pregnant, Ron landed a union job at one of the city's biggest slaughterhouses, and his pay more than doubled, enabling them to move into a two-bedroom apartment on the corner of Dubuc and Des Meurons Streets. Then the couple had a scare. When she was in the latter stages of her pregnancy, Janet developed a serious case of toxemia—a pregnancy-related form of high blood pressure that, untreated, can be harmful to the fetus. Her doctor recommended that she have her labor and delivery induced.

On 22 August 1965, some four weeks before her projected due date, Janet was admitted to St. Boniface Hospital. During his wife's labor, Ron sat in the visitor's lounge nervously awaiting the outcome. After several hours, a nurse came and announced that everything had gone fine and that he was the father of identical twins. In his relief and excitement at hearing that Janet and the babies were alive and well, Ron failed to take in anything else. So as he hurried through the doorway toward the nursery to see his children, he was brought up short by a smiling nurse who called out to him, "Boy or girl?"

"I don't know!" Ron called back. "I just know there's *two* of 'em!"

They named the twins Bruce and Brian. They were so similar in appearance that people could not tell them apart, but Janet and Ron, like the parents of most identical twins, could soon distinguish the children easily. Bruce, the elder of the two by twelve minutes, had been born slightly underweight and as a result had had to stay in the hospital a few days to be fattened up. But by the time he joined his twin brother at home, it was clear that he was the more active child, tending to writhe and wriggle and to wake in the night with greater frequency than his brother Brian, a peaceful, less rowdy baby. Both bore a striking resemblance to Janet, with their upturned noses and small round mouths.

By the time the boys were six months of age, Janet felt like an old hand at pacifying, feeding, and changing them. Ron had received another raise, and the family moved to a still bigger and nicer place to live—an actual house on Metcalfe Street, not far from their former apartment. Life seemed to be shaping up beautifully for the young family.

Which is what made it so unsettling when, shortly after the twins were seven months old, Janet noticed that they seemed to be in distress when they urinated. At first she thought it was just the wet diapers that made them cry; then she noticed that even after a diaper change they would scream and complain. She examined their penises and noticed that their foreskins seemed to be sealing up at the tip and making it difficult for the boys to pass water. She took the babies to see her pediatrician, who explained that they were suffering from a condition called phimosis. It was not rare, he said, and was easily remedied by circumcision. After talking about it with Ron, Janet agreed to have the children circumcised at St. Boniface Hospital.

The operations were scheduled for the morning of 27 April, but because Ron was working the late shift at the slaughterhouse, he and Janet decided that he should drive the kids in to be admitted the night before. Apart from the normal concern any parent would feel on the eve of such an operation, Ron and Janet felt no particular trepidation about the circumcisions. Nor should they have. St. Boniface was an excellent, fully modern general teaching hospital. Housed in a seven-story building, it had seven hundred beds, a cardiac care unit, and a children's hospital where, in the mid-1960s, some 2,600 babies were delivered annually and roughly a thousand circumcisions performed each year, all without mishap.

"We weren't worried," Janet says. "We didn't know we had anything to worry about."

Ordinarily, pediatricians experienced in circumcisions performed the procedure at St. Boniface Hospital, but on the morning of 27 April 1966 the usual attending physician, for reasons lost to history, was not available when the Reimer twins were scheduled for their operations. The duty fell to Dr. Jean-Marie Huot, a forty-six-year-old general practitioner.

When a nurse was dispatched to collect the first of the children, it was pure happenstance that she lifted baby Bruce from the bassinet first.

With the baby fixed and draped on the operating table, Dr. Max Cham, the anesthesiologist, administered gas to put Bruce to sleep. (Though newborns were routinely circumcised without anesthesia, a child of eight months, like baby Bruce, could not be operated on while conscious.) Sources differ slightly on what happened next. Court papers later filed against the surgeon, hospital, and three attending nurses refer to an "artery clamp" that was used to secure the piece of foreskin that was meant to be cut away. An artery clamp, however, would be a most unusual choice for such a procedure. According to Dr. Cham, with whom I spoke in the winter of 1997, Dr. Huot used the standard Gomco clamp. Designed specifically for circumcisions, the clamp is used to prevent excessive bleeding: the foreskin is stretched over a bell-shaped metal sheath; a round clamping device then closes over the stretched foreskin and compresses it against the bell, squeezing the foreskin and thus making it blood-free for excision by scalpel.

Regardless of which clamp was used, it is not in doubt that Dr. Huot elected to use not a scalpel to cut away Bruce's foreskin, but a Bovie cautery machine. This device employs a generator to deliver an electric current to a sharp, needlelike cutting instrument, which burns the edges of an incision as it is made, sealing the blood vessels to prevent bleeding—a quite superfluous consideration if Huot had indeed used a Gomco clamp, and a dangerous one, since it would bring perilously close to the penis a current that could be conducted by the metal bell encasing the organ. If, at the same time, the current to the needle were to be turned up almost to the maximum, the results could be cataclysmic.

According to the later testimony of operating room personnel, the electrocautery machine was turned on, and the hemostat dial, which controlled the amount of heat in the needle, was set at the minimum. Dr. Huot lowered the needle and touched it to Bruce's foreskin. Subsequent testing of the machine revealed that it was in proper working order. Whether through temporary mechanical malfunction, user error, or some combination of the two, the needle failed to sever the flesh on the first pass. The hemostat control was turned up. Once again the instrument was applied to the foreskin; again it failed to cut. The cautery machine's current was increased. The needle was once again brought into contact with the foreskin.

"I heard a sound," recalls Dr. Cham, "just like steak being seared."

A wisp of smoke curled up from the baby's groin. An aroma as of cooking meat filled the air.

A urologist was quickly summoned. On duty that morning was Dr. Earl K. Vann. He cleared the instruments and inspected the organ. It appeared oddly blanched in color. He felt the penis with his gloved hand and noticed that it had an unusual firmness. Vann took a probe and attempted to pass it through the urinary meatus—the hole at the end of the penis. The probe would not pass through. Vann told the operating room personnel that he would have to perform an emergency suprapubic cystotomy to place a catheter and thus enable the baby to pass urine. He made an incision below Bruce's belly button, then threaded a length of tubing into the incision, through the muscle wall, and into the bladder. This was sewn into place. A bag to catch the child's urine was affixed to the free end of the catheter. The baby was then wheeled out to the burn ward.

It was decided not to attempt to circumcise his twin brother.

On nights when Ron worked the late shift, the Reimers' normal routine was for Janet to prepare dinner, which they would eat together when Ron got home from work shortly after midnight. They would talk about their day, maybe watch a little TV, and often not make it to bed until two or three in the morning. They'd usually sleep until noon or one. They were sleeping on the morning of 27 April when the phone rang.

Janet answered. It was the hospital calling.

"They said to come in and see the doctor," Janet recalls. "They said there was a slight accident, and they needed to see us right away." Ron took the phone and asked the person on the other end of the line what was going on. "They just said they wanted to see us," Ron says. "They didn't say there was anything wrong."

But Ron and Janet could tell by the person's tone of voice that something unusual was happening. They dressed and headed out to their car. Opening their front door, they discovered that the city, which for some weeks had been in the full delicious flood of early spring, had been hit by a freak blizzard. The pathway to the curb was completely obliterated by snow; the car was buried up to its bumpers. Flakes continued to sift down thickly from a bleached sky.

Ron dug the car out, and they began the slow journey through streets clogged and snarled with snowbound traffic. Five blocks north on St. Mary's Road, then a right turn onto Tache Avenue and the eight blocks up to the hospital. Over the car radio they heard that the airport had been closed down. Seven inches were expected to fall over the course of the day. Already the weathermen were proclaiming it one of the worst blizzards in the city's history. Longtime residents would recall the storm clearly more than thirty years later.

Having finally made it the one mile from their house to St. Boniface Hospital, Ron and Janet rushed inside, only to wait in the doctor's office for what seemed a very long time. Dr. Huot entered. In a businesslike voice he told the Reimers that there had been an accident while circumcising baby Bruce.

"What do you mean, an accident?" Janet said.

Dr. Huot said that Bruce's penis had been burned.

"I sort of froze," Janet recalls. "I didn't cry. It was just like I turned to stone." When she finally gathered her wits enough to speak, Janet found herself asking if they had also burned her *other* child.

"No," Dr. Huot replied. "We didn't touch Brian."

Ron and Janet asked to see their injured baby right away. The doctor said that Bruce was recovering from a surgical procedure to install a catheter. The Reimers were told not to worry, that they could see the child tomorrow. They collected their uninjured son, Brian, and drove home through the steadily falling snow.

The next day Ron and Janet returned to the hospital. Dr. Vann took them to see the baby. Janet's first glimpse of her son is a memory that even three decades later causes her face to drain of blood. Standing over Bruce's bassinet in the burn unit, she looked at his penis—or what was left of it.

"It was blackened, and it was sort of like a little string. And it was right up to the base, up to his body." To Ron the penis looked "like a piece of charcoal. I knew it wasn't going to come back to life after that."

Nevertheless, Janet asked the urologist, "Will it still grow, and he'll just have a *little* penis?"

The doctor shook his head. "I don't think so. That's not the way it works."

Over the next few days, baby Bruce's penis dried and broke away in pieces. It was not very long before all vestiges of the organ were gone completely.

Bruce remained in the hospital while Ron and Janet watched a parade of the city's top local specialists examine him. The doctors gave little hope. Phallic reconstruction, a crude and makeshift expedient even today, was in its infancy in the 1960s—a fact made plain by the plastic surgeon, Dr. Desmond Kernahan, when he described the limitations of a penis that would be constructed from flesh farmed from Bruce's thigh or abdomen. "Such a penis would not, of course, resemble a normal organ in color, texture, or erectile capability," Kernahan wrote in his consultation report. "It would serve as a conduit for urine, but that is all." Even that was optimistic, according to Dr. M. Schwartz, a urologist who also examined the child: "Insofar as the future outlook is concerned," he wrote, "restoration of the penis as a functional organ is out of the question." Dr. G. L. Adamson, head of the Department of Neurology and Psychiatry at the Winnipeg Clinic, evaluated Bruce's projected psychological and emotional future. "One can predict," Adamson wrote, "that he will be unable to live a normal sexual life from the time of adolescence: that he will be unable to consummate marriage or have normal heterosexual relations, in that he will have to recognize that he is incomplete, physically defective, and that he must live apart."

Pediatrician Dr. Harry Medovoy was also called in to consult on the case. Though Medovoy had spent his entire career practicing in Manitoba, he had an international reputation. He was a member of the editorial board of the American journal *Pediatrics* and founder of a children's hospital at the Winnipeg Health Sciences Center, which bears his name today. Though he was a relentless booster of Canadian medicine, it was Medovoy's opinion that the child should be seen at one of the major American medical centers. He recommended the Mayo Clinic, a mere half-day's train ride away in Rochester, Minnesota. Thus, upon Bruce's release from the hospital on 7 June—six weeks after he was first admitted to St. Boniface—Ron and Janet took him on the train to Rochester.

At the Mayo Clinic the baby was examined by a team of doctors. They recommended that Bruce have an artificial phallus constructed at some time shortly before he began school. Like the Winnipeg doctors, the Mayo Clinic physicians explained that phalloplasties were by no means foolproof: they required multiple surgeries through childhood, and the cosmetic and functional results were not promising.

Ron and Janet could hardly believe that this was all the Mayo Clinic doctors could offer them. They wondered why they had bothered to go to the expense and trouble of coming all the way to this famous medical center merely to hear what they had heard back in Canada.

Feeling that they had now exhausted all their options, Ron

and Janet returned to Winnipeg and tried to reconcile themselves to raising a son who, no matter how successful the phalloplasty, "must live apart."

The *Winnipeg Free-Press* and its rival, the *Tribune,* soon got
wind of the story. The newspapers each ran an article about a
child whose penis was burned off at St. Boniface Hospital. The
press did not print the Reimers' name, however, so Ron and
Janet were able to keep secret from their neighbors the dreadful
accident that had befallen their child. When Janet accepted
invitations from other young mothers in the neighborhood to
come over for coffee, she sat silently while the others happily
traded information about their babies. Only when she got
home did she burst into tears and wail, "I hate you, God!" Her
taciturn husband, typically, permitted himself no such outpour-
ing of emotion. Ron had once tried to confide in a couple of
friends at work about the accident, but the guys joked about it.
"I stopped talking to those people," Ron says. "I stopped talking to everybody, pretty much." It only added to the young couple's misery that Brian's phimosis had long since cleared up by
itself, his healthy penis a constant reminder that the disastrous
circumcision on Bruce had been utterly unnecessary in the first
place.

The twins' first birthday, on 22 August 1966, passed in
gloom for Ron and Janet. By January they felt like prisoners
in their house. They could not even go out together to see a
movie (if they had felt so inclined), since they were afraid to
hire a baby-sitter who might gossip about the tragedy. By
February, Ron began to wake in the middle of the night from
dreams that he was strangling Dr. Huot.

Then on a Sunday evening in mid-February—some ten

months after Bruce's accident—Ron and Janet saw something that jolted them from their despondency. Their small black-and-white TV happened to be tuned to the Canadian Broadcasting Corporation's popular current affairs program *This Hour Has Seven Days*, where a man identified as Dr. John Money was a guest. A suavely charismatic individual in his late forties, bespectacled and with the long, elegantly cut features of a matinee idol, Dr. Money was talking about the wonders of gender transformation taking place at Johns Hopkins Hospital in Baltimore.

Today, with the subject of transexual surgeries a staple of daytime talk shows, it is difficult to imagine just how alien the concept seemed on that February evening in 1967. Fifteen years earlier, in 1952, a spate of publicity had attended the announcement by American ex-GI George Jorgensen that he had undergone surgical transformation to become Christine. That operation, performed in Denmark, had been roundly criticized by American hospitals, which refused to perform the surgeries. The subject had faded from public view—until now, when Johns Hopkins announced that it had not only performed two male-to-female sex changes, but had established the world's first clinic devoted solely to the practice of converting adults from one sex to the other. The driving force behind the renowned hospital's adoption and promotion of the controversial procedure was the man who now appeared on the Reimers' TV screen: Dr. John Money.

The name rang a distant bell for Ron and Janet. Shortly after Bruce's accident, one of the Winnipeg plastic surgeons had said that he had mentioned Bruce's case to a leading sex researcher at a medical meeting in the United States; the man had suggested that Ron and Janet raise Bruce as a girl. The doctors at the Mayo Clinic had also said something to Ron and Janet about a man in Baltimore who could help them raise Bruce as a girl. While the Mayo Clinic doctors had not themselves recommended the procedure, they had said that the Reimers might like to get a second opinion. At the time, Ron and Janet had not even considered the idea of a sex change. Or so they had thought. As they watched Dr. Money on television, they realized that the idea had never completely left them; it had lodged in the backs of their minds, as Ron puts it, "like a seed that had been planted." Now, as they watched and listened to Dr. Money speak, it was as if that seed had grown and burst into full flower.

It was his confidence that was most striking. Even under the pressure of the staring television cameras and live studio audience, Dr. Money's words, tinged with a highly cultured, British-sounding accent, issued forth with uncanny fluency. He did not stumble over a single syllable, even when the show's interviewer—a bulldoglike young man named Alvin Davis—asked pointedly why psychiatrists were "so opposed" to the practice that Dr. Money was promoting.

"Well," Money said, "I suppose it's a self-evident fact that there are many people who feel that this is not the psychiatric way to treat these patients, since the usual definition of psychiatry is in terms of psychotherapy and the talking treatment. However, there are a small group of people who, like myself, believe that it's thoroughly justified in an attempt to constantly increase our ability to help human beings and to see exactly what the outcome is when, let's say, twenty or thirty people can be followed for five to ten years after having received this kind of treatment."

"But isn't it a fact," Davis said, "that a homosexual will come to you and say, 'I want to be castrated.' And then *you* will make the judgment—or you and a board, a panel at Johns Hopkins will make the judgment—about whether to castrate that person?"

"Yes," Dr. Money said, mildly. "If you want to state it that way, it's true."

"Not only to castrate that person," Davis continued, his voice taking on the rising tone of a prosecutor, "but to inject hormones into the person and virtually change the person—*not* into a female, but into a male with female parts. Aren't you arrogating to yourselves certain decisions that not only psychiatrists don't want to have, but perhaps God doesn't want to have?"

"Well," Dr. Money said, the flicker of a smile underlining the martini-dry sarcasm in his tone, "would *you* like to argue on God's side?"

"No," Davis said. "I would like to know whether *you* believe God doesn't belong in this."

"Well," Money replied, returning to his tone of unflappable calm, a tone ever so slightly shaded by patient condescension, "I'm not sure that's really a particularly relevant question— although I'm aware that many would. May I," he continued, "give you the answer of the group of ministers in Baltimore who were interrogated by the press at the time of the announcement in the papers there? The thirteen of them agreed that in terms of the magnitude of the problem—especially in terms of its magnitude in the lives of the people concerned—that this was ethically justifiable as an attempt to help them. There was one person who withheld an answer until a later date, and that was a representative of the Roman church."

"Why isn't the work being done here in Canada?" Davis demanded to know. And he repeated his earlier query: "And why are so many psychiatrists here so opposed to it?"

"Oh," Money said, almost languidly, "I would think for the same reason that there tends to be a traditionalism in most places. I don't need to tell you that in many branches of medicine, science—or even housekeeping or farming—there is a tendency to hang on to the past, to cling to the past."

"And *you're* the pioneer?" Davis asked.

"Well," Dr. Money said, "perhaps in a small way."

At this point the camera cut from Dr. Money and his questioner to a blond woman who walked out onto the set. Dressed in a narrow skirt, high heels, and a matching close-fitting jacket, she took a seat in the chair across from the two men. A close-up shot revealed that her round, pretty face was expertly made up, in the style of the mid-1960s, with heavy eyeliner, mascara, and foundation, her mouth thickly painted with lipstick.

"This is Mrs. Diane Baransky," the show's announcer said. "Until four years ago, her name was Richard."

Ron and Janet gaped at the TV screen. It was their first glimpse, ever, of a transexual. It was one thing to hear Dr. Money talk about sex change in the abstract; it was another to see it with your own eyes. Ron and Janet could hardly believe it. If they hadn't been told that Mrs. Baransky was born a man, they would never have guessed it. Even *knowing* it, it was hard to believe. She looked like an attractive, even *sexy* woman. The way she moved, walked, sat—even her voice, despite an ever so slight huskiness, had the timbre of a woman's as she said hello to her host and fellow guest.

After a few preliminary questions from Davis, Dr. Money spoke up, deftly seizing the reins of the interview.

"Diane," he said, "I think people would be extremely interested if you could give us a short sketch of the difference that it makes to have had this procedure—to compare the old life with the new."

"Well, there is a tremendous difference," Mrs. Baransky said. "It's a way of finding yourself. You actually fit into society, you're more accepted in a more normal society." She explained that the discrepancy between her anatomic self as a male and her inward sense of herself as a female had been a trial to her growing up. "As a teenager—or being young—when you're different from anybody else, it's very hard." Becoming a woman, Mrs. Baransky explained, had solved all her problems of being teased and "singled out." Until her sex change, she had felt completely alone. Now she was accepted as a woman and had recently married her husband, a fellow hairdresser. "I was different," she said. "I was never complete. I was neither a man nor a woman."

"And now you feel complete as a woman?" Davis asked.

Her response was unequivocal: "Oh, yes, definitely. Yes. Completely—body and mind."

The audience was then invited to ask questions. It was near the end of the segment that a young man asked the question that had been forming in Janet's mind. He asked about "the other group of sex patients" whom Dr. Money treated—newborn babies with what Dr. Money had earlier called "unfinished genitals," babies whose private parts were neither male nor female at birth. In replying to this question, Dr. Money explained that he and his colleagues at Johns Hopkins could, through surgery and hormone treatments, make such children into whichever sex seemed best, and that the child could be raised happily in that sex. "The psychological sex in these circumstances," as Dr. Money put it, "does not always agree with the genetic sex nor with whether the sex glands are male or female."

Despite the big words and the rapidity with which Dr. Money spoke them, Janet and Ron caught their meaning. Dr. Money was saying that the sex a baby was born with didn't matter; you could convert a baby from one sex to the other.

Janet turned to Ron. "I think I should write to this Dr. Money," she said.

Ron agreed. When the segment ended a few minutes later, Janet wrote a letter to Dr. Money describing what had happened to Bruce. Dr. Money's reply was prompt. He expressed great optimism about what could be done for the Reimers' baby at Johns Hopkins and urged them to bring the child to Baltimore without delay.

After so many months of grim predictions, bleak prognoses, and hopelessness, Dr. Money's words, Janet says, felt like a balm. "Someone," she says, "was finally *listening*."

2

≡

Dr. Money was indeed listening. In a sense, Janet's cry for help was one that he might have been waiting for his entire professional life.

At the time the Reimer family's plight became known to him, John Money was already one of the most respected, if controversial, sex researchers in the world. Born in 1921 in New Zealand, he had come to America at the age of twenty-five, received his Ph.D. in psychology from Harvard, then joined Johns Hopkins, where his rise as a researcher and clinician specializing in sexuality was meteoric. Fifteen years after joining Johns Hopkins, he was already widely credited as the man who coined the term *gender identity* to describe a person's inner sense of himself or herself as male or female. He was also known as the world's undisputed authority on the psychological ramifications of ambiguous genitalia and was making headlines around the world for his establishment of the pioneering Johns Hopkins clinic for transexual surgeries.

As his unflappable appearance on *This Hour Has Seven Days* would suggest, Money was also a formidable promoter of his ideas. "He's a terribly good speaker, very organized, and very persuasive in his recital of the facts regarding a case," says Dr. John Hampson, a child psychiatrist who, with his wife, Joan, coauthored a number of Money's groundbreaking papers on sexual development in the mid-1950s. "I think a lot of people were envious. He's kind of a charismatic person, and some people dislike him."

Money's often overweening confidence actually came to him at some cost. His childhood and youth in rural New Zealand had been beset by anxieties, personal tragedies, and early failure. The son of an Australian father and an English mother who belonged to the Brethren church, he was a thin, delicate child raised in an atmosphere of strict religious observance—or what he would later derisively call "tightly sealed, evangelical religious dogma." His sense of intellectual superiority developed early. On his first day of school at age five, he was set upon by bullies and took refuge with a female cousin in the girls' play-shed, where boys would not be caught dead. "Having not measured up as a fighter," Money would later write, "I was set on the pathway of outwitting other kids by being an intellectual achiever. That was easier for me than for most of them."

Money's childhood difficulties were compounded by his vexed relationship with his father. Six decades later he would write with barely controlled venom of this father, portraying him as a brutal man who heartlessly shot and killed the birds that infested his fruit garden, and administered to his four-year-old son an "abusive interrogation and whipping" over a broken window. This incident, Money wrote, helped establish his lifelong rejection of "the brutality of manhood."

Money was eight years old when his father died of a chronic

kidney ailment. "My father died without my being able to forget or forgive his unfair cruelty," Money wrote. Not told of his father's death until three days after seeing him carried off to the hospital, Money's shock was compounded by the experience of being informed by an uncle that now *he* would have to be the man of the household. "That's rather heavy duty for an eight-year-old," Money wrote. "It had a great impact on me." As an adult, Money would forever avoid the role of "man of the household." After one brief marriage ended in divorce in the early 1950s, he never remarried, and has never had children.

After his father's death, Money was raised in an exclusively feminine atmosphere by his mother and spinster aunts, whose anti-male diatribes also had a lasting effect on him. "I suffered from the guilt of being male," he wrote. "I wore the mark of man's vile sexuality"—that is, the penis and testicles. In light of Money's future fame in both adult and infant sex change, his next comment has an unsettling tenor: "I wondered if the world might really be a better place for women if not only farm animals but human males also were gelded at birth."

A solitary adolescent with a passion for astronomy and archaeology, Money also harbored youthful ambitions as a musician, a goal doomed to disappointment once Money realized that he would never be more than a skilled amateur. As an undergraduate at Victoria University, in the New Zealand capital city of Wellington, Money discovered a new passion into which he rechanneled his thwarted creativity: the science of psychology. Like so many students drawn to the study of the mind and emotions, Money's interest in the discipline was in large part as a means for solving certain troubling questions about himself. His first serious work in psychology, his master's thesis, concerned "creativity in musicians," in which, Money writes, "I began to investigate my relative lack of success in comparison with that of other music students."

His decision soon after that to narrow his studies to the psychology of sex had a similarly personal basis. Having departed sharply from his parents' faith, Money grew increasingly to react against what he saw as the repressive religious strictures of his upbringing. The academic study of sexuality, which removed even the most outlandish sexual practices from moral considerations into the "pure" realm of scientific inquiry, was for Money an emancipation. From his twenties on, he would be a fierce proselytizer for sexual curiosity and exploration. By the mid-1970s, with the sexual revolution in full rampage, Money would step out publicly as a champion of open marriage, nudism, and other more rarefied manifestations of the culture's sexual unbuttoning. "There is plenty of evidence that bisexual group sex can be as personally satisfying as a paired partnership, provided each partner is 'tuned in' on the same wavelength," he wrote in his book *Sexual Signatures*. Elsewhere, he has described his own private life as casual and eclectic—"a give-and-take of sexual visitations and friendly companionships with compatible partners, some women, some men."

Reveling in his role as "agent provocateur of the sexual revolution" (as the *New York Times* dubbed him in 1975), Money rarely missed an opportunity to spread his gospel of sexual emancipation: extolling the heightened pleasures of sex under a black light to a student after a speaking engagement at the University of Nebraska; appearing in court as an expert witness to defend the 1973 pornographic film *Deep Throat*, which he praised as a "cleansing" movie that would help keep marriages together; penning op-ed pieces for the *New York Times* in which he called for a "new ethic of recreational sex." A patient treated by Money in the 1970s for a rare endocrine disorder recalls the psychologist once casually asking him if he'd ever experienced a "golden shower." A sexually inexperienced youth at the time, the patient did not know what Money was talking about. "Getting pissed on," Money airily announced with the twinkling, slightly insinuating smile with which he liked to deliver such deliberately provocative comments.

Convinced that embargoes on certain words promoted prudery, Money inserted the words *fuck*, *cock*, and *cunt* into his regular conversation with colleagues and patients. Dr. Fred Berlin, a professor of psychiatry at the Johns Hopkins School of Medicine and a colleague who considers Money one of his most important mentors, defends Money's penchant for sexual outspokenness. "Because he thinks it's important to desensitize people in discussing sexual issues," Berlin says, "he will sometimes use four-letter words that others might find offensive. Perhaps he could be a little more willing to compromise on that, but John is an opinionated person who isn't looking necessarily to do things differently than the way he's concluded is best."

While Money's conclusions about the best approach to sexual matters merely raised eyebrows in the mid-1970s, they provoked outrage at the dawn of the more conservative 1980s, when Money ventured into areas of which even some of the most adventurous sexual explorers were leery. In 1986, Money published *Lovemaps,* an exhaustive study of such practices as sadomasochism, coprophilia, amputation fetishes, autostrangulation, and various other behaviors that he called, not perversions, but "paraphilias," in an effort to destigmatize and decriminalize them. The topic of pedophilia became a particular interest, and one that Money took obvious delight in publicly espousing.

"A childhood sexual experience," he explained to *Time* magazine in April 1980, "such as being the partner of a relative or of an older person, need not necessarily affect the child adversely." He granted an interview to *Paidika*, a Dutch journal of pedophilia, which carries ads for the North American Man-Boy Love Association and other pro-pedophile groups.

"If I were to see the case of a boy aged ten or twelve who's intensely attracted toward a man in his twenties or thirties, and the relationship is totally mutual, and the bonding is genuinely totally mutual, then I would not call it pathological in any way," he told the journal, and added, "It's very important once a relationship has been established on such positive and affectionate grounds that it should not be broken up precipitously." In 1987, Money wrote an admiring foreword to an unusual volume published in Denmark entitled *Boys and Their Contacts with Men*. By Dutch professor Theo Sandfort, the book presented what purported to be verbatim testimonials of boys as young as eleven years old rhapsodically describing the delights of sex with men as old as sixty. "For those born and educated after the year 2000," Money wrote, "we will be their history, and they will be mystified by our self-important, moralistic ignorance of the principles of sexual and erotic development in childhood." Money concluded his foreword with the proclamation "It is a very important book, and a very positive one."

Money's response to criticism for the public airing of such views was always to launch counterattacks of his own, ridiculing his critics for their adherence to an outmoded sexual Puritanism. In an autobiographical essay included in his 1985 book of collected writings, *Venuses Penuses*, Money dubbed himself a "missionary" of sex, proudly proclaiming, "It has not been as easy for society to change as it had been for me to find my own emancipation from the 20th-century legacy of fundamentalism and Victorianism in rural New Zealand."

Money's experimental, taboo-breaking attitude to sex found its echo in the way he pursued his professional research career. Eschewing the more trammeled byways of sex

research, Money deliberately sought out exotic corners of the
field. He found just such a relatively undiscovered realm of
human sexuality in 1948, while in the first year of study for
his Ph.D. in psychology at Harvard. In a tutorial called Field-
work and Seminar in Clinical Psychology, Money was presented with the case of a fifteen-year-old genetic male born
not with a penis, but with a tiny, nublike phallus resembling a
clitoris. At puberty, the boy had developed breasts. It was
Money's first exposure to hermaphroditism—also known as
intersexuality—a term of classification for a variety of birth
anomalies of the internal and external sex organs. Often
described in lay terms as a condition of being half-man, half-
woman, the syndrome derives its name from a combination of
the names of the Greek gods of love, Hermes and Aphrodite,
and occurs as often as one in two thousand births (by some
estimates). The symptoms vary from the extreme manifesta-
tion of a genetic female born with a penis-sized clitoris and
fused labia resembling a scrotum, to a male whose genital
resemblance to a girl at birth is so total that his true biological sex is not suspected until puberty when "she" fails to menstruate—to anything in between.

Money was fascinated by hermaphroditism and wrote his
doctoral dissertation on the subject. Until then the syndrome
had been studied almost solely from a biological perspective.
Money approached it from a psychological angle, investigat-
ing the mental and emotional repercussions of growing up as
anatomically neither boy nor girl. His thesis, entitled "Hermaphroditism: An Inquiry into the Nature of a Human Paradox," was completed in 1952 and led to his invitation to join
Johns Hopkins, where the world's first and largest clinic for
studying and treating intersexual conditions had been established. The clinic's director, pioneering pediatric endocrinologist Lawson Wilkins, teamed Money with two married psy-

chiatrists, Drs. Joan and John Hampson, to study the mental and emotional makeup of the intersexual patients treated in the clinic. The three researchers made up the newly created Psychohormonal Research Unit.

Over the next six years, Money and the Hampsons studied some 131 intersexuals ranging in age from toddlers to adults. Money (who was lead investigator and author of the team's published reports) claimed to observe a striking fact about intersexes who had been diagnosed with identical genital ambiguities and chromosomal makeups but raised in the opposite sex from one another: more than 95 percent of them reportedly fared equally well psychologically whether they had been raised as boys or girls. Money called these groupings of patients "matched pairs" and said they were proof that the primary factor determining an intersexual child's gender identity was not biology, but rather the way the child was raised. He concluded that these children were born wholly undifferentiated in terms of their psychological sex and that they formed a conception of themselves as masculine or feminine solely through rearing.

This theory was the foundation on which Money based his recommendation to Johns Hopkins surgeons and endocrinologists that they could surgically and hormonally steer intersexual newborns into whichever sex, boy or girl, they wished. Such surgeries would range from cutting down enlarged clitorises on mildly intersexual girls to full sex reversal on intersexual boys born with undeveloped penises. These conversions to girlhood were foreordained by the state of surgical technology: it was easier for surgeons to construct a synthetic vagina than to create an artificial penis. Money's only provisos were that such "sex assignments" and reassignments be done within the first two and a half years of life (after which time, Money theorized, a child's psychosexual orientation ceased to be as malleable) and that once the sex had been decided upon, doctors and parents never waver in their decision lest they risk introducing fatal ambiguities into the child's mind.

By providing a seemingly solid psychological foundation for such treatments, Money had offered physicians a relatively simple surgical solution to one of the most vexing and emotionally fraught conundrums in medicine: how to deal with the birth of an intersexual child. "One can hardly begin to imagine what it's like for a parent when the first question—'Is it a boy or a girl?'—results in a response from the physician that they're just not sure," says Dr. Fred Berlin. "John Money was one of those folks who, years ago, before this was even talked about, was out there doing his best trying to help families, trying to sort through what's obviously a difficult circumstance."

Money, however, was not interested chiefly in intersexes. As he stated as early as his Harvard thesis, he recognized the scientific worth of intersexes primarily as what he called "experiments of nature"—as a cohort of research subjects who could shed light on the question of sexual development in *normal* humans—who could, in fact, resolve one of the longest-running debates in science; namely, whether it is primarily nature or nurture that shapes our sexual sense of self. It was in his first published papers at Johns Hopkins that Money generalized the theory of psychosexual neutrality at birth from hermaphrodites to include *all* children, even those born without genital irregularity.

"From the sum total of hermaphroditic evidence," he wrote in 1955, "the conclusion that emerges is that sexual behavior and orientation as male or female does not have an innate, instinctive basis. In place of a theory of instinctive masculinity or femininity which is innate, the evidence of hermaphroditism lends support to a conception that, psychologically, sexuality is undifferentiated at birth and that it becomes differentiated as masculine or feminine in the course of the various experiences of growing up." In short, Money was advancing a view that human beings form a sense of themselves as boy or girl according to whether they are dressed in blue or pink, given a masculine or feminine name, clothed in pants or dresses, given guns or Barbies to play with. Many years later, Money would describe how he arrived at some of his more radical theories about human sexual behavior. "I frequently find myself toying with concepts and working out potential hypotheses," he mused. "It is like playing a game of science fiction."

While Money's theory of human newborns as total psychosexual blank slates may strike a contemporary reader as science fiction, such was not the case in the mid-1950s, when it was met with almost universal acceptance by clinicians and scientists—an acceptance not difficult to understand in the context of the time. Explanations for sex differences had been moving toward a nurturist view for decades. Prior to that, the pendulum had been pointing in the naturist direction—thanks to the discovery at the end of the nineteenth century of the so-called male and female hormones, testosterone and estrogen. The discovery of these chemical-based internal secretions had led biologists to proclaim the riddle of sex differences solved: testosterone was the masculinizing agent; estrogen, the feminizing. They confidently predicted that male homosexuals would be discovered to possess an excess of the "female" hormone in their bloodstream and a deficiency of the "male" hormone. Minute analysis of the urine and blood of adult homosexual men, however, revealed no such hormonal imbalances. Under the microscope, a straight and a gay man's internal secretions are identical. Other experiments meant to show the hormonal basis of sexual identity also failed, and as the failures mounted, enthusiasm for a biological explanation of sexual differences gradually waned. Simultaneously, the first half of the twentieth century and the advent of Freud and modern psychology saw a rapid increase in social learning models for human behavior. Against this background, the Johns Hopkins team's conclusions that sexual identity and orientation were solely shaped by parents and society fit perfectly into an intellectual zeitgeist in thrall to behaviorist theories. Nor did it detract from the papers' reception that they carried the imprimatur of Johns Hopkins Hospital, one of the premier medical research institutions in the world.

The Johns Hopkins team's 1955 intersex papers were proclaimed instant classics and won that year's Hofheimer Prize from the American Psychiatric Association. The Hampsons soon left Johns Hopkins for Washington State University and by 1961 had drifted out of gender identity research. As a result, Money alone became heir to the award-winning papers' reputation. And as sole director of the Psychohormonal Research Unit (after Lawson Wilkins's death in 1962), he was also the lone beneficiary of the unit's success. In 1963 Money was awarded a grant of $205,920 from the National Institutes of Health—a considerable sum in early-1960s dollars, but merely the first of several NIH grants that would sustain Money and his unit for the next thirty-five years. In 1965 he served as Mead Johnson visiting professor of pediatrics at the University of Buffalo Children's Hospital, and was awarded the Children's Hospital of Philadelphia Medal "for contributions to the study of the psychological development of children." A year later he would begin to garner fame outside the academic realm when he finally succeeded in persuading Johns Hopkins to establish the clinic for the treatment and study of adult transexuals.

Money had been galvanized by transexualism since 1952, when the revelations about Christine Jorgensen first hit the press. In Jorgensen's case, Money saw tantalizing proof of his theory that environment, not biology, determines psychological sex, for here was a person born with apparently normal male biological makeup and genitals whose inner sense of self had differentiated as female—in direct contradiction to his chromosomal, gonadal, hormonal, reproductive, and anatomic sex. What greater evidence could there be that gender identity is determined not by biology but by environment? Determined to study such individuals in the greatest number possible, Money set out to get Johns Hopkins into transexual research and treatment, which was still a repellent idea for the majority in the American medical establishment.

In his campaign to establish Johns Hopkins as the first hospital in America to embrace transexual surgeries, Money knew that he would first have to bring on board a respected medical man. (Money himself was a psychologist and did not possess a medical degree of any kind.) He turned first to Dr. Howard Jones, the Johns Hopkins gynecologist who had perfected the surgical techniques for sex assignment on Money's infant intersexual subjects. "I can recall," Jones says, "that for a number of months, maybe even *years,* John kept raising the question of whether we shouldn't get into the transexual situation." While Jones was interested in experimental medicine (he would eventually leave Johns Hopkins for the University of Virginia where he would found the nation's first in vitro fertilization clinic), he was resistant to the idea of performing elective castrations and genital reconstruction on adults.

But Money was persistent. He turned for help to Dr. Harry Benjamin. The acknowledged grandfather of transexual study in America, Benjamin had for the previous ten years been quietly referring transexual patients to doctors in Casablanca and Morocco for sex change surgery. Money enlisted three of Benjamin's postoperative transexuals to come to Johns Hopkins and meet with Jones and pediatric endocrinologist Milton Edgerton. Eventually Jones and Edgerton were convinced. "John finally marshaled enough evidence," as Jones puts it, "to indicate that this was something that maybe should be done." Fittingly enough, Money was given the job of naming the new clinic for adult transexual surgeries. He dubbed it the Gender Identity Clinic.

The first complete transexual surgery at Johns Hopkins was performed by Dr. Jones on 1 June 1965, when a New Yorker named Phillip Wilson became Phyllis Avon Wilson. But it still remained for Johns Hopkins to sell the idea to the American public. While some members of the sex change committee argued for keeping the existence of the clinic quiet, Money pushed for a preemptive strike and argued in favor of creating a press release that would circumvent leaked rumors about what the team had done. Money's argument prevailed, and he helped concoct a press release with the hospital's public relations department. The statement was issued on 21 November 1966. Money later revealed that a strategic decision had been made to issue the press release to the *New York Times* alone. The prestige of the *Times*, the Johns Hopkins team hoped, would set the tone for all other media coverage. "The plans," Money later wrote, "worked out exactly as hoped."

The *Times* treated the revelations with none of the scandalized outrage that had greeted the Jorgensen case in 1952. The front-page story used verbatim quotations from Gender Identity Clinic chairman John Hoopes, culled directly from the Johns Hopkins press release, and presented the procedure as a humane and effective solution to an intractable psychosexual problem. Similarly approving stories followed in all three news weeklies, *Time, Newsweek,* and *U.S. News & World Report.* In April 1967 *Esquire* magazine published an exhaustive feature on the Johns Hopkins clinic, in which Money was admiringly quoted. Indeed, of all the coverage in late 1966 and early 1967 of Johns Hopkins' pioneering foray into transexual surgery, by far the hardest edged was CBC's *This Hour Has*

Seven Days, in which Alvin Davis sharply challenged Money on the ethics and efficacy of switching people's sex. Except for the single stinging rejoinder ("Would *you* like to argue on God's side?"), Money had refused to rise to the bait, and thus, for his fellow Gender Identity Clinic committee members, set the standard for how to handle direct attacks. Money's calm, judicious performance was a masterpiece of public relations, and all the more impressive to those who knew the ferocity with which, in ordinary life, he responded to even the mildest opposition to his opinions.

As Money himself would admit in an essay written in 1990, "In the practice of my psychohormonal research, I do not suffer fools gladly." This was an understatement. The psychologist's violent reactions to intellectual challenge were legendary. "John was unusually brilliant," says Dr. Donald Laub, a pioneer in adult transexual surgical techniques who has known Money for thirty years. "He may be the smartest person I've ever met. He was so smart that it was a *problem*—because he knew everybody *else* was dumb." By all accounts, Money had no compunction about letting others know his low opinion of their intellectual firepower. "Even when John asked for feedback, what he was looking for was agreement," says Dr. Howard Devore, a psychologist who earned his Ph.D. under Money in the Psychohormonal Research Unit in the mid-1980s. Should that agreement fail to be forthcoming, Money was never afraid to let his displeasure be known. As early as the mid-1950s, Money had a reputation for tantrums among his coworkers, underlings, and students that preceded him throughout the academic world.

"Every center that I trained at after [Johns Hopkins]," says Devore, "when people saw on my résumé that I had worked with John Money, they would ask me to comment, off the record, what it was like working with him and was he 'as bad as people say?' I was just amazed at how consistent his world-wide reputation actually was. And frankly, John didn't do that much to hide it. I once saw him stand up at an academic meeting and shout a presenter down because he didn't agree with what she was saying."

By February 1967—when Ron and Janet Reimer first saw John Money on television—his reputation was for all intents and purposes unassailable. Dr. Benjamin Rosenberg, himself a leading psychologist who specialized in sexual identity, says that Money was "the leader—the front-runner on everything having to do with mixed sex and hermaphrodites and the implications for homosexuality and on and on and on."

Money's reach and influence throughout the academic and scientific world would help to define the scientific landscape for decades to come—indeed, to the present day: many of his students and protégés, trained in his theories of psychosexual differentiation, have gone on to occupy the top positions at some of the most respected universities, research institutions, and scientific journals in the country. His former students include Dr. Anke Ehrhardt, now a senior professor at Columbia University; Dr. Richard Green, director of the Gender Identity Clinic in London, England; Dr. June Reinisch, who for years was head of the famed Kinsey Institute; and Dr. Mark Schwartz, director of the influential Masters and Johnson Clinic.

On the clinical side, Money's influence was perhaps even more remarkable. His theories on the psychosexual flexibility at birth of humans form the cornerstone of an entire medical speciality—pediatric endocrinology. Professor Suzanne Kessler, in her 1998 book, *Lessons from the Intersexed*, suggests that Money's views and their implications for the treatment of ambiguously sexed babies form among physicians "a consensus that is rarely encountered in science."

There was, however, at least one researcher in the mid-1960s who was willing to question John Money. He was a young graduate student fresh from the University of Kansas.

The son of struggling Ukrainian Jewish immigrant parents, Milton Diamond, whom friends called Mickey, was raised in the Bronx, where he had sidestepped membership in the local street gangs for the life of a scholar. As an undergraduate majoring in biophysics at the City College of New York, Diamond had become fascinated by the role hormones played in human behavior. Seeking a place to do graduate work, he chose Kansas, where anatomist William C. Young (famous for his hallmark studies of the 1930s on the role of hormones in the estrus cycle) ran a laboratory. In a stroke of serendipity, Diamond's arrival in Kansas in the fall of 1958 coincided with the time when a trio of researchers on Young's staff—Charles Phoenix, Robert Goy, and Arnold Gerall—stood on the brink of a discovery about the sex-differentiating role of hormones that would change the science and study of sexual development forever.

Disillusionment with earlier hormone studies had led many sex researchers, including Young's team, to shift their focus from the role played by hormones in the mature organism to the role played by hormones in the womb. Working from guinea pig studies done two decades earlier by Soviet sex researcher Vera Dantchakoff, the Kansas team sought to learn the role played by the hormones that bathe a developing fetus's brain and nervous system. Earlier researchers had shown that, in humans, in the early stages of gestation, the male and female fetus's internal and external sex organs are identical to one another. Between six and eight weeks, however, changes start to take place. If the fetus's cells bear the male (XY) chromosome, the fetal gonads differentiate as testicles, which begin to pump out testosterone. This prenatal androgen is the agent that masculinizes the developing fetus's external genitals—turning the undifferentiated genital tubercle into a penis, causing the open genital sinus to fuse along the midline and form the scrotum, into which the testicles descend—and at the same time masculinizes the internal reproductive system by spurring the growth of the seminal ducts (another testicular secretion suppresses growth of the rudimentary female internal structures). If, on the other hand, the fetus bears the female (XX) chromosome, the gonads develop as ovaries, no testosterone is produced, in the absence of which the external genitals and internal anatomy differentiate as female, the genital tubercle develops as a clitoris, the genital sinus remains open and becomes the entrance to the vagina, and the internal structures develop as fallopian tubes and uterus.

The question for the Kansas team was whether these prenatal hormonal effects on the anatomy were mirrored in the brain. To find out, they set about creating a cohort of hermaphrodite guinea pigs by injecting large doses of testosterone into the wombs of pregnant mothers. When exposed to testosterone at a critical stage in fetal development, the female guinea pigs were born, as expected, with clitorises enlarged to the size of penises. The researchers then set out to learn if the masculinization of a treated female's anatomy was matched by a corresponding masculinization of her sexual behavior.

In observing the treated females as they grew from childhood to maturity, the team noticed something extraordinary. Not only did the treated females demonstrate an increased physical activity distinct from that of their untreated sisters, they also did not, in the presence of normal males, present their hindquarters for sexual penetration in the normal female in-heat posture known as lordosis. Instead, the testosterone-treated females (even those that showed no clitoral enlargement) attempted to mount their untreated sisters.

I spoke with team member Robert Goy, shortly before his death in 1999, about the breakthrough moment of his research career. His voice was charged with an excitement that suggested he had just made the discovery the night before. "We couldn't schedule tests fast enough," he told me. "We were testing every night—night after night after night—and getting data, and analyzing it, and reanalyzing it."

Milton Diamond was in the thick of the research, performing adjunct experiments on the pregnant mothers to learn what, if any, influence the testosterone had on their functioning. Having come to Kansas hoping to learn something new and interesting about the action of hormones on behavior, Diamond found himself present at one of the most significant biological breakthroughs in sex research of the twentieth century.

There was concern among members of the team about how their professor, William Young, would react to the results. They knew him to be an adherent of the theories of psychosexual neutrality advanced just four years earlier by John Money's team at Johns Hopkins. "Young was a great follower of John Money and the Hampsons," Goy told me. "He had been thinking all this time that the organizing principle for sexual behavior was experience. So his world was shaken by these results. But he was wonderfully adaptable, and the truth was more important to him than anything else. It's very unusual in a scientist. Most scientists fall in love with their own ideas and theories, and you can't shake them out of it. Will Young wasn't like that."

In fact it was Young who settled the debate that flared among the research team members when it came time to write up the results. Unsure precisely how to label the behavior of the treated female guinea pigs—the team toyed with calling it "masculine mimicry" or "pseudodifferentiation"—they were overruled by Young, who told them they had discovered not the role played by prenatal testosterone in creating a *simulation* of masculine behavior, but masculine behavior itself. Accordingly, Young advised the team to state unequivocally that they had discovered, in the fetal guinea pig, the *organizing principle* for adult masculine sexual behavior.

"Young was an anatomist," Goy explained, "and if you understand the way anatomists use the term *organization,* it makes that choice of word inevitable. Anatomists believe that the organs of the body are organized by a set of tissues that are differentiated in a special way and combined so that they carry out a definite function or malfunction of that organ. And that's the way he used the word *organization.* He meant that all of the tissues underlying sexual behavior—whether peripheral structures, brain tissues, blood, or muscles—are organized into a whole; and that that organization is imposed by exposure to hormones before birth; and that that organization is either masculine or feminine. And he believed that we had discovered the principle that organizes the tissues in a masculine form."

Still, when the team came to write up their results, which would appear in a 1959 issue of the journal *Endocrinology,* Young urged caution in how directly they should extrapolate their experimental animal work to sexual differentiation in humans—largely out of Young's respect for Money's work with the Hampsons. The team agreed to soften their statements on the applicability of their research to humans. "We said there may be some way that the guinea pig picture will 'complement' or 'supplement' the human picture by accounting for 'discrepancies,'" Goy said.

Not everyone in the lab was satisfied with that decision. The youngest member, Mickey Diamond, felt that Young and the others were being too cautious in failing to link their animal findings directly to the human situation. "I believe in evolution," Diamond says, chuckling. "I didn't see any reason that human beings would be different from other mammals in that regard." He felt so strongly that when he was applying for a research grant in his final year at Kansas and was required to submit an original paper, he decided to write an essay taking on Money and the Hampsons' theory of psychosexual neutrality at birth.

In that paper, entitled "A Critical Evaluation of the Ontogeny of Human Sexual Behavior," Diamond rejected outright the Johns Hopkins team's theory. Citing the guinea pig findings, Diamond described as "specious" a theory that said man is "completely divested of his evolutionary heritage," and stated that prebirth factors "set limits" on how far culture, learning, and environment can direct gender identity in humans. Marshaling evidence from biology, psychology, psychiatry, anthropology, and endocrinology to argue that gender identity is hardwired into the brain virtually from conception, the paper was an audacious challenge to Money's authority (especially coming from an unknown graduate student at the University of Kansas).

Addressing the theory about the psychosexual flexibility of intersexes, Diamond pointed out that such individuals had experienced "a genetic or hormonal imbalance" in the womb, and he argued that even if human hermaphrodites *could* be steered into one sex or the other as newborns (as Money claimed), this was not necessarily evidence of their gender neutrality at birth. It might simply suggest that the organization of their nervous systems and brains had undergone in utero a similar ambiguous organization as their genitals. In short, they had an inborn neurological capability to go both ways—a capability, Diamond hastened to point out, that genetically normal children certainly would not share. As for transexuals, who showed no observable anatomic ambiguity of sex, Diamond postulated that they, too, might possess an as yet undiscovered biological condition that hardwired their brains to a program opposite to the evidence of their bodies—a possibility that Diamond was able to back up with evidence from no less an authority than Dr. Harry Benjamin himself, who had recently reported that in forty-seven out of eighty-seven of his patients, he "could find no evidence that childhood conditioning" was involved in their conviction that they were living in the wrong sex.

Had he known of it at the time, Diamond might also have drawn upon an obscure paper in the foreign literature for his critique—a paper that had questioned the Johns Hopkins team's protocols for intersex treatment some six years earlier. In a 1959 edition of *The Canadian Psychiatric Association Journal*, three Toronto physicians, Dr. Daniel Cappon, Dr. Calvin Ezrin, and Dr. Patrick Lynes, had pointed out serious flaws in the Hopkins team's statistical and research methods. "[T]hese workers," the Canadians wrote, "failed to relate the physical and psychological wholes of the person and only compared component parts without submitting these comparisons to mathematical validation." In conducting their own research on a cohort of seventeen intersexual patients, the Canadian doctors took precautions that the Johns Hopkins team had not. To prevent subjective tainting of their results, the Canadians split their research team in two: one to study the patients from an endocrinologic perspective, the other to study the patients from a psychological perspective. For comparative purposes, the Canadian team also carried out research on a control group of nonhermaphrodites, as well as on a series of homosexuals and transvestites.

The team's results showed that it was dangerous indeed to suppose that no link existed between an intersexual child's biological makeup and its gender identity; that in fact the status of the chromosomes, gonads, or hormones might predispose a hermaphrodite child to identify more with one sex than the other in adulthood. Stating that the Johns Hopkins team had based its recommendations to surgeons on "shaky theory," the Canadians had expressed particular unease about the recommendation that males born with tiny or nonexistent penises should, without exception, be castrated and converted into girls. Such sex-changed children, the Canadians had warned, "were liable to be brought up tragically incongruously with the main somatic sex."

The Canadian team's findings would have made a strong addition to Diamond's exhaustive theoretical critique, but he did not learn of the paper's existence until after his own was published (at which point he began to cite it in his own papers). "The Canadian paper got lost somewhere," Diamond says. "It just died. I think it was maybe Hopkins compared to Podunk." But in 1965, Diamond's paper was published in a high-profile, well-respected American journal, the *Quarterly Review of Biology*, where it could not be missed—least of all by John Money, considering that the *Quarterly Review* was at that time published out of Johns Hopkins.

I was sitting with Diamond in his cluttered, windowless office on the campus of the University of Hawaii Medical School as he reminisced about these origins of his thirty-year-long scientific debate with John Money. It was June of 1997, just two months after Diamond and Sigmundson's "John/Joan" paper had delivered a blow to his old rival. A mild-mannered sixty-four-year-old with frizzy graying hair and beard, Diamond was clearly exhausted from fielding the unending stream of phone calls, faxes, and letters from both reporters and fellow scientists requesting more information about, or an interview with, John/Joan. Dressed in a pale blue overlaundered T-shirt riddled with holes, a pair of jeans, and battered running shoes, Diamond told me that professors at the University of Hawaii are "paid in sunshine." His putty-colored pallor suggested that he had not been drawing his full wages. Diamond had, in fact, spent the majority of his thirty years in Honolulu doing experiments or hunched over his computer in the tiny office he calls his "cave," pumping out more than one hundred journal articles and eight books on sexuality. On the wall beside him was tacked a snapshot of his four daughters; on the messy desk in front of him were heaped papers, books, open journals, and boxed sets of both Robert Johnson and Bach tapes.

Diamond insists that he bore John Money no personal animus at the time of writing his 1965 article and that his intent was not to embarrass him. He says that his paper had merely been an effort to advance the field of knowledge in the time-honored scientific tradition of assertion and challenge. Diamond points out that after the article's publication, he actually made an overture to Money, suggesting that they collaborate on an article. Though he recognized that they stood on opposite sides of the nature-nurture debate, Diamond believed this was precisely why their collaboration would be of particular value. He shakes his head and smiles at the naïveté that compelled him, a mere graduate student, to suggest a collaboration with one of the leading scientists in the field—a scientist whom, furthermore, he had just publicly challenged in a leading journal. "I really believed that it was an intellectually good thing to do," Diamond says. Money evidently felt otherwise. "His attitude was, Why should I do anything with *you*?" Diamond says. "Who knows *you*?" Diamond admits that he was not completely surprised by the reaction. "I had challenged his theory, which he took as an argument against *him*. Which it wasn't."

Yet even a scientist less thin-skinned than John Money might have been stung by the calm, relentless logic of Diamond's critique—which, near the end, raised the most rudimentary Science 101 objection to the unquestioning acceptance of Money's theory of psychosexual neutrality in normal children. "To support [such a] theory," Diamond wrote, "we have been presented with no instance of a normal individual appearing as an unequivocal male and being reared successfully as a female." And Diamond had added: "If such an individual is available he has not been referred to by proponents of a 'neutrality-at-birth' theory. It may be assumed that such an individual will be hard to find."

Hard—but not, as events transpired, impossible. For it was just one year and eight months after Diamond threw down this gauntlet in the *Quarterly Review of Biology* that Dr. John Money received a letter from a young mother in Winnipeg, Canada, describing the terrible circumcision accident that had befallen one of her identical twin baby boys.

3

=

RON AND JANET REIMER made their first trip to Johns
Hopkins in early 1967, shortly after seeing Dr. Money on TV.
The young couple—aged twenty and twenty-one respectively—were awestruck by the vast domed medical center
dominating the top of a rise on Baltimore's Monument Street.
Dr. Money's Psychohormonal Research Unit was located in
the Henry Phipps Psychiatric Clinic, a gloomy Victorian
building tucked away off a back courtyard. The unit's offices,
located on the fourth floor, were reached by way of a rickety
turn-of-the-century elevator. Money's own inner sanctum
(where most of his meetings with the Reimers would take
place over the next eleven years) reflected the psychologist's
eccentric tastes in interior decoration. Furnished with a
couch, Oriental rugs, and a profusion of potted plants, the
room also featured brightly colored afghans thrown over the
backs of armchairs, a collection of carved aboriginal sculptures of erect phalluses, vaginas, and breasts on a mantel, and

a collection of primitive blowguns, darts, and masks hanging on the walls. The Reimers had certainly never seen anything like this before, but Dr. Money, with his smoothly confident, professional manner—not to mention the diplomas on his wall—made the Reimers feel that they were, finally, in the best possible hands. "I looked up to him like a god," says Janet. "I accepted whatever he said." And what Dr. Money had to say was exactly what the Reimers ached to hear.

In his many published versions of this first interview, Money has recounted how he spelled out to the young couple the advantages of sex reassignment for their baby—"using nontechnical words, diagrams, and photographs of children who had been reassigned." He explained to Ron and Janet that their baby could be given a perfectly functional vagina—"adequate for sexual intercourse and for sexual pleasure, including orgasm." He also explained to them that although their child would not, if changed into a girl, be able to bear children, she would develop psychologically as a woman and would find her erotic attraction to men. As a married woman she would be perfectly capable of adopting children of her own.

What is not clear from Money's written accounts of this meeting is whether Janet and Ron, whose education at the time did not go beyond ninth and seventh grades, respectively, understood that such a procedure was in fact purely experimental—that while Money and his colleagues at Johns Hopkins had performed sex reassignments on hermaphrodite children, no such infant sex change had ever been attempted on a child born, like their Bruce, with normal genitals and nervous system. Today Ron and Janet say that this was a distinction they did not fully grasp until many years later. The crucial point they gleaned from Dr. Money was his conviction that the procedure had every chance for success. "I see no reason," Janet recalls him saying, "that it shouldn't work."

Money's eagerness to begin seemed evident in his recounting of the interview almost ten years later. "If the parents stood by their decision to reassign the child as a girl," he wrote in *Sexual Signatures*, "surgeons could remove the testicles and construct feminine external genitals immediately. When she was eleven or twelve years old, she could be given the female hormones."

If Dr. Money seemed to be in a hurry, he was. He explained to Ron and Janet that they would have to make up their minds quickly. For according to one of the finer points of his theory, the *gender identity gate*—Money's term for that point after which a child has locked into an identity as male or female—comes at two and a half to three years of age. Bruce was now nineteen months. "The child was still young enough so that whichever assignment was made, erotic interest would almost certainly direct itself toward the opposite sex later on," Money wrote, "but the time for reaching a final decision was already short."

Ron and Janet, however, were not prepared to have Bruce immediately admitted to the hospital. They needed time to decide on something as momentous as having their child undergo a surgical sex change. They told Dr. Money that they would have to go home and think about it. Janet says that he made no secret of his impatience with the delay. Upon their return to Winnipeg, the couple received letters from him urging them to reach a final decision. "He wrote in a letter that we were 'procrastinating,'" Janet recalls, "but we wanted to move slow because we had never heard of anything like this."

Back home, Ron and Janet canvassed opinions. Their pediatrician recommended against such drastic treatment and stuck by his earlier advice that Ron and Janet wait until the child was of preschool age before beginning the long process of phalloplasty. Janet's mother, Betty, was inclined to trust the expert from Baltimore but had no real opinion of her own. Ron decided not even to bring it up to his parents since he felt sure they would be against it.

Finally Ron and Janet realized that only they could decide the fate of their child. They alone were the ones living with the reminder, at each diaper change, of his terrible injury. Janet saw the benefits of changing their son into a daughter. "I didn't know much back then," she says, "and I thought women were the gentler sex. Mistakenly. I have since learned that women are the hard-core knockabout tough guys. *Men* are the gentler sex, by far, from my experience. But I thought, with his injury, it would be easier for Bruce to be raised as a girl—to be raised gently. He wouldn't have to prove anything like a man had to."

Ron, too, could see the benefits of changing Bruce's sex. "You know how little boys are," Ron says. "*Who can pee the furthest?* Whip out the wiener and whiz against the fence. Bruce wouldn't be able to do that, and the other kids would wonder why." And then, of course, there was the entire question of Bruce's sex life. Ron could not even imagine the humiliations and frustrations that would entail. As a girl and woman, though, Bruce wouldn't face all that, Ron reasoned. If what Dr. Money told them was true, she could live a normal life, she could get married, she could be happy.

Within days of their return from Baltimore, Ron and Janet stopped cutting the baby's hair, allowing the soft, light brown locks to curl down past the ears. Janet used her sewing machine to turn his pajamas into girlish granny gowns. Their son had become, for Ron and Janet, their daughter. Dr. Money had counseled them, when deciding what to call their new daughter, to select a name beginning with the same letter as her former name and to avoid calling her after any female family members with whom her identity could become confused. Janet, following Dr. Money's instructions, called her new baby daughter Brenda Lee.

There was, of course, still one more step to take. That summer, Ron and Janet left Brenda's twin brother, Brian, with an aunt and uncle, then flew back to Baltimore with their daughter. Now twenty-two months old, she was still within the window that Money had established as safe for infant sex change. On Monday, 3 July 1967, Brenda underwent surgical castration in a gynecologic operating room at Johns Hopkins Hospital. The surgeon was Money's Gender Identity Clinic cofounder, Dr. Howard Jones. Today Jones says he can recall few specifics about the case. He says that all decisions regarding reassignment of sex were the responsibility of Money and pediatric endocrinologist Dr. Robert Blizzard.

"My chief interest was the physical situation and the surgical potential," Jones says. "Was the patient healthy and able to withstand the operation?—all that kind of stuff. The case was pretty well worked up before I ever got involved." For Jones, the surgery on Brenda Reimer was like the routine castrations he had been performing on hermaphrodite babies over the previous twelve years—and apparently Johns Hopkins Hospital viewed the operation the same way. Officials of the hospital have declined all comment on the case, but a Johns Hopkins public relations person, JoAnne Rodgers, told me in the winter of 1998, "In all surgeries that were considered, in the sixties, to be experimental, there were protocols in place to have those approved by appropriate committees and boards." Dr. Jones cannot recall that the hospital convened any special committee or board in the case of Bruce Reimer's historic conversion to girlhood.

The main procedure was a bilateral orchidectomy—removal of both testicles. As Jones's operating room notes reveal, the baby, under general anesthesia, was placed on his back on the operating table, each foot secured in a stirrup so that the groin was exposed for the doctors. Three clamps were placed on the scrotum, and two incision lines were drawn on either side of the midline. With a pair of scissors, Dr. Jones cut away the demarcated scrotal flesh in a strip 1.5 centimeters long to lay bare the testicles and seminal vesicles within. With a scalpel, Jones cut away both the right and left testicles, then used a length of catgut thread to tie off the cord and vessels that in adulthood would have carried sperm to the severed urethra.

In closing the scrotum, Dr. Jones then fashioned a rudimentary exterior vagina using the remaining scrotal skin, which he pulled up from its lower edge to meet the top edge of the incision and sewed in a manner that left the scrotum not as a single empty sack, but as two symmetrical flaps. "A rolled piece of gauze covered with telfa was then placed in the midline to effect a midline furrow leaving constructed labia majora on either side," Jones's operating room note concludes.

Ron and Janet say that by the time they decided to have their baby undergo clinical castration, they had eradicated any doubts they might have had about the efficacy of the treatment. This was a crucial turnabout since according to Dr. Money it was a "vital consideration" that the parents of a sex-reassigned child harbor no doubts that could weaken the child's identification as a girl and woman.

Whether Dr. Money himself was able to eradicate his own doubts about the child's future development is debatable. In a letter he wrote on 28 August 1967, more than a month after Brenda's sex change surgery, his tone admitted of considerable caution regarding the child's prognosis. This was perhaps to be expected, since the letter was addressed to the Winnipeg lawyer whom Ron and Janet had hired to sue St. Boniface Hospital and the doctor who had botched the circumcision.

"The reassignment of a baby's sex is usually undertaken only in cases of a birth defect of the genitalia," Money wrote. "Then one usually expects that the child's psychosexual differentiation will be congruous with the sex of rearing. In any given case, however, it is not possible to make an absolute prediction."

And indeed, by the summer of 1967, when Bruce Reimer underwent his castration, Dr. Money had special reason to be particularly reluctant to make an "absolute prediction" about the patient's future psychosexual development. Two years earlier he had undertaken to discover if the findings of the Kansas team about the masculinizing effects on behavior of prenatal testosterone in guinea pigs could be observed in humans. Under Money's direction, one of his graduate students, Anke Ehrhardt, had studied a group of ten girls, ranging in age from three to fourteen, who had been subjected to excesses of testosterone in the womb when their pregnant mothers had taken a synthetic steroid called progestin to prevent threatened miscarriage. Like the guinea pigs in the Kansas team's study, nine of the ten girls had been born with masculinized genitals—an oversized clitoris and in some cases partially fused labia. As interviews with the children and their parents revealed, all nine of those girls demonstrated what Money and Ehrhardt called (in an article published six months before Bruce Reimer's castration) "tomboyishness." This, the authors explained, included marked preferences for "masculine-derived" clothes and "outdoor pursuits," a "strong interest in boys' toys" (these included guns and toy soldiers), a "high incidence of interest and participation in muscular exercise and recreation," and a "minimal concern for feminine frills, doll play, baby care, and household chores."

≡

Central to Dr. Money's program for the sex assignment of hermaphrodites was his edict that the children, when very young, know nothing of their ambiguous sexual status at birth. Money put the same stricture into effect with baby Brenda Reimer. "He told us not to talk about it," Ron says. "Not to tell Brenda the whole truth and that she shouldn't know she wasn't a girl."

It was shortly after the Reimers' return from Baltimore, and not long before the twins' second birthday, when Janet first put Brenda in a dress. It was a special dress that Janet had sewn herself, using the white satin from her own wedding gown. "It was pretty and lacy," Janet recalls. "She was ripping at it, trying to tear it off. I remember thinking, Oh my God, she knows she's a boy and she doesn't want girls' clothing. She doesn't want to be a girl. But then I thought, Well, maybe I can *teach* her to want to be a girl. Maybe I can train her so that she wants to be a girl."

Ron and Janet tried their best to do just that. They furnished her with dolls to play with; they tried to teach her to be neat and tidy; and they tried, whenever possible, to reinforce her identity as a girl. So when, for instance, the twins had just turned four, and Brian was watching Ron shave and asked if he could shave, too, Ron gave him an empty razor and some shaving cream to play with. When Brenda also clamored for a razor, Ron refused. "I told her girls don't shave," Ron says. "I told her girls don't have to." Janet offered to put makeup on Brenda, but Brenda didn't want to wear makeup.

"I remember saying, 'Oh, can I shave, too?'" David says of this incident, which forms his earliest childhood memory of life as Brenda. "My dad said, 'No, no. You go with your mother.' I started crying, 'Why can't *I* shave?'"

Brian says that the episode was typical of the way their parents tried to steer him and his sister Brenda into opposite sexes—and how such efforts were inevitably doomed to failure. "I recognized Brenda as my sister," Brian says. "But she never, ever acted the part."

Today, with the twins having rejoined each other on the same side of the gender divide, the stark physical differences between them eerily testify to all that David has been through. When David first introduced me to Brian in the summer of 1997, I instinctively assumed that the man who took my hand in a firm grip was an *older* brother, so different did this balding, dark-bearded, bearlike man look from his youthfully thin, smooth-faced brother. It was only when I looked a little closer at Brian's face and recognized the startling familiarity of the eyes, nose, and distinctively shaped mouth that I realized I was meeting David's identical twin, and that he was in fact the *younger* of the two (albeit by a scant twelve minutes).

As children, their physical differences were, if less pronounced, equally deceptive. Photographs of them as preschoolers show a pair of exceptionally attractive children: a puppy-eyed little boy with a crew cut, and a slim, brown-eyed girl with wavy chestnut hair framing a face of delicate prettiness. However, by all accounts of family, teachers, guidance clinic workers, and relatives, this illusion of two children of opposite sexes disappeared the second Brenda moved, spoke, walked, or gestured.

"When I say there was nothing feminine about Brenda," Brian laughs, "I mean there was *nothing* feminine. She walked like a guy. Sat with her legs apart. She talked about guy things, didn't give a crap about cleaning house, getting married, wearing makeup. We both wanted to play with guys, build forts and have snowball fights and play army. She'd get a skipping rope for a gift, and the only thing we'd use *that* for was to tie people up, whip people with it. She played with *my* toys: Tinkertoys, dump trucks. This toy sewing machine she got just sat." That is, David recalls, until the day when Brenda, who loved to take things apart to see how they worked, sneaked a screwdriver from her dad's tool kit and dismantled the toy.

Enrolled in Girl Scouts, Brenda was miserable. "I remember making daisy chains and thinking, If this is the most exciting thing in Girl Scouts, forget it," David says. "I kept thinking of the fun stuff my brother was doing in Cubs." Given dolls at Christmas and birthdays, Brenda simply refused to play with them. "What can you *do* with a doll?" David says today, his voice charged with remembered frustration. "You *look* at it. You *dress* it. You *undress* it. Comb its hair. It's boring! With a car, you can drive it somewhere, *go* places. I wanted cars." Brenda also wanted toy guns. Once, around age eight, she went to the store to buy an umbrella. Waiting in line to pay, she saw a nearby display of toy machine guns. After a moment's hesitation, she put down the umbrella and bought one of the guns. At age ten, Brenda would prove to be a crack shot with the pellet rifle Ron and Janet bought for Brian—a rifle in which, ironically enough, Brian himself evinced little interest.

Brenda had always tried to co-opt Brian's toys and clothes—a habit that would invariably initiate fights. "There were knock-down-drag-out wrestling matches all the time," Janet says. "Brian was a weakling compared to Brenda. She was wiry. More often than not, Brenda won. Poor Brian felt so bad getting beat up by a girl."

Ron and Janet were troubled by Brenda's masculine behavior, but having been admonished by Dr. Money not to entertain any doubts about their daughter, they felt that to do so would only increase the problem. Instead they tried to focus on those moments when Brenda's behavior *could* be construed as stereotypically feminine. "She could be sort of feminine sometimes, when she wanted to please me," Janet says. "She'd be less rough, keep herself clean and tidy, and help a little bit in the kitchen."

In her letters to Dr. Money describing Brenda's progress, Janet made sure to emphasize those moments so that the psychologist would know that Janet and Ron were doing everything they could to implement his plans. She also informed Money of their daughter's masculine leanings, but the psychologist assured her that this was mere "tomboyism." This was an explanation that Janet found comforting, and she would cling to it for many years to come. "I have seen all kinds of women in my life," she says, "and some of them, you'd swear they were men. So I thought, Well, maybe it won't be a problem, because there are lots of women who aren't very effeminate. Maybe it could work. I *wanted* it to work."

Ron's and Janet's parents were struck by Brenda's behavior. "When a girl would come to play with her," says Ron's mother, Helen, "she would not play like a girl, and then she would say to her mother that she wanted the girl to go home."

"I noticed it when she had that fight with the boy across the street," says Janet's mother, Betty. "This boy tried to beat her up. And Brenda beat back."

Janet's uncle Johnny and aunt Evelyn were also unable to ignore certain realities about their niece. They might have surmised that Brenda was simply imitating Brian, but they knew better. They knew Brian particularly well because they were the ones who had baby-sat him for the three weeks while Ron, Janet, and Brenda were in Baltimore for Brenda's operation. Without his sister around, Brian had been a quiet, gentle, sensitive boy—quite unlike the little terror who was tearing up Ron and Janet's home with Brenda. Johnny and Evelyn formed the private opinion that, if anything, *Brenda* was the leader of the pair, and it was Brian who followed her lead into boyish mayhem and mischief. "She was the instigator," Johnny says. Neither Johnny nor Evelyn ever voiced this to Ron and Janet, of course. "We were trying to go along with this," Evelyn explains. "We were not going to start looking for trouble."

Brenda, meanwhile, was having her own doubts. "You don't wake up when you're four and a half years old, look at the clock, and say, 'Yup, I feel like a boy,' " David explains. "You're too young." At the same time, he says he knew something was amiss, even before he fully understood the concept of boy and girl. "I thought I was very similar to my brother. It's not so much me being a guy, it's more that we were *brothers*. It didn't matter that I was in a dress."

Brian didn't question his sister's boyish ways until they went off to school. "I was in grade one or two," he says, "and I saw all these other girls doing their thing, combing their hair, holding their dolls. Brenda was not like that. Not at all." At that time Brenda voiced the ambition to be a garbage man. "She'd say, 'Easy job, good pay,' " Brian explains. "I thought it was kinda bizarre—my *sister* a garbage man?" Brian would finally grow so perplexed with his sister's unconventional behavior that he went to his mother about it. "Well, that's Brenda being a tomboy," Janet told him, which he accepted.

It was not an explanation that Brenda's schoolmates were prepared to accept, however. Upon entering kindergarten at Woodlawn, a small school near their house, Brenda became the object of instant ridicule from both boys and girls. "As you'd walk by, they'd start giggling," David recalls. "Not one, but almost the whole class. It would be like that every day. The whole school would make fun of you about one thing or another."

"It started the first day of kindergarten," Janet says. "Even the teacher didn't accept her. The teacher knew there was something different."

She did indeed. Contacted twenty-six years later, the twins' kindergarten teacher, Audrey McGregor, said she had never seen a girl like Brenda before or since. At first glance the child looked like the thousands of other girls who have passed through McGregor's classroom, but there was a rough-and-tumble rowdiness, an assertive, pressing dominance, and a complete lack of any demonstrable feminine interests that were unique to Brenda in McGregor's experience. And there was something else. McGregor mentions an incident that occurred shortly after the school year began. "A female classmate of Brenda's came up to me," McGregor recalls, "and she asked, 'How come Brenda stands *up* when she goes to the bathroom?' "

Ever since setting out to toilet train the twins, Janet had been grappling with Brenda, trying to convince her daughter not to stand and face the toilet bowl when she peed. No amount of coaxing seemed to work. Janet had mentioned the problem to Dr. Money, who had assured her that it was common for girls to insist on standing up to urinate and that the problem would correct itself in time. It had not. For Janet, Brenda's stubborn insistence on standing created a housekeeping nightmare, since Brenda's urine stream, which shot out almost perpendicular to her body from her severed urethra, splashed all over the back of the toilet seat. As for any suggestion that Brenda's stubborn insistence on standing up to urinate indicated that the treatment was not working—this was not, Janet says, something she could afford to believe.

Kindergarten teacher McGregor, unschooled in Money's theories of child development, formed a quite different opinion about Brenda. "She was more a *boy*," McGregor says, "in the *nature* of things." Furthermore, McGregor was convinced that Brenda herself, on some unconscious level, knew this. "I don't think she *felt* she was a little girl," the teacher says.

McGregor's surmise was correct. Plunged into the sexually polarized world of school, Brenda now knew there was something seriously different about her. "You know generally what a girl is like," David says, "and you know generally what a guy is like. And everyone is telling you that you're a girl. But you say to yourself, I don't *feel* like a girl. I liked to do guy stuff. It didn't match. So you figure, Well, there's something *wrong* here. If I'm supposed to be like this girl over here, but I'm acting like this guy, I guess I gotta be an *it*."

Brenda's personal difficulties were obvious in her functioning in the classroom. On her year-end Kindergarten Inventory of Skills, she was rated unsatisfactory in category after category: Social Living, Work Habits, Listening Skills, Speaking Skills, Reading Skills. The school threatened to hold Brenda back to repeat kindergarten. Janet complained to Dr. Money during a follow-up visit to Johns Hopkins. Dr. Money responded by giving the child an IQ test. Over two days, his research assistant, Nanci Bobrow, administered the Wechsler Intelligence Scale (the standard IQ test). Brenda scored in the low 90s, which placed her in the middle 50 percent of the population, indicating an average intelligence. Three weeks later Dr. Money sent the results to Brenda's school. In an accompanying letter he painted a portrait of Brenda as a girl whose problems were temporary and well on the way to clearing up once she got over what he called her "playful negativism," which was the result of "the bad emotional situation created by her early hospitalizations."

"In such a case as the present one," he concluded, "I very strongly favor promotion, because the degree of under achievement observed is a function of an emotional interference-factor which will definitely not improve by retaining the child at the kindergarten level."

The school authorities in Winnipeg, upon receipt of

Dr. Money's letter, reversed their recommendation, and in September 1971, Brenda was advanced to first grade at a new school called Minnetonka.

Brenda's problems only got worse. On 29 October, less than two months after Brenda started first grade, her teacher, Sharyn Froome, filed a report with the district's Child Guidance Clinic. "I have had an extremely hard time interesting Brenda in any games or activities," wrote Froome, who saw Brenda's negative behavior as anything but "playful." Describing her simply as "very negativistic," and noting the child's total isolation from her peers, Froome wrote that Brenda "has been doing just the opposite of anything the other children do."

Child Guidance Clinic worker Joan Nebbs was among those who observed Brenda's functioning at this time. "Her mother would send her to school very clean and cutely dressed, in little fancy tops and things like that," Nebbs recalls. "She was quite fine-featured, with curly hair, and was a very pretty child with big brown eyes. It was her manner more than anything else that got in the way. She was always grubby. She'd always just been fighting with the kids and playing in the dirt. Brenda was *really* a rough little kid. She didn't want to sit down with a book. She'd rather play knock-'em-down-shoot-'em-up cop games." Nebbs says that Brenda sometimes tried to play with girls, but with little success. "She'd be trying to organize the girls to do things her way—trying to be the boss. She'd want them to play cowboys and Indians, chasing everyone around, general mayhem—and they didn't want any part of that."

Ron and Janet, who had hoped to keep Brenda's medical history confidential, had no choice but to recognize that that would be impossible. After repeated queries from both the school and the Child Guidance Clinic for information about Brenda that might throw light on her academic and social difficulties, Ron and Janet signed a confidentiality waiver authorizing their local pediatrician, Dr. Mariano Tan, to contact the Child Guidance Clinic.

"I hope you will keep this letter strictly confidential," Dr. Tan wrote to the clinic's director. "Both of these children have been under my care since Oct., 1966. They are identical twins—both *male*—however, because of an unfortunate accident during circumcision on Bruce (now Brenda), the penis was amputated." Tan went on to explain about Brenda's sex change at Johns Hopkins.

The revelations in Tan's letter seemed to explain, for both the clinic and the school, much about Brenda Reimer. "I just agreed it was a girl until I heard different," says Brian's first grade teacher, June Hunnie. "Once we knew the *background,* we thought to ourselves, Well, no wonder. What can you do to have a child sit down and quietly concentrate on classwork if there's all this horrible stuff going on in the background? It's impossible."

Indeed it was—at least for Brenda. At the end of that school year, Minnetonka informed Ron and Janet that while Brian would be promoted to the next grade in the fall of 1972, Brenda (despite Dr. Money's sanguine predictions) would have to remain behind.

4

≡

O<small>N</small> 28 D<small>ECEMBER</small> 1972, four months after Brenda Reimer began her second attempt at first grade, John Money unveiled his "twins case."

The occasion was the annual meeting of the American Association for the Advancement of Science in Washington, D.C. There Money delivered to a capacity crowd of over one thousand scientists, feminists, students, and reporters the first speech in a two-day series of talks devoted to "Sex Role Learning in Childhood and Adolescence." The symposium, held in the Ambassador Ballroom of the Shoreham Hotel, featured an impressive roster of leading researchers in the field of sexual development. Only Money's appearance at the meeting would make headlines, however—thanks to the remarkable case he cited that morning, a still fuller account of which (he informed his audience) could be found in his book *Man & Woman, Boy & Girl* (coauthored with Anke Ehrhardt)—a book that happened to have been published, in an early example of cross-promotional marketing, the very day of Money's appearance at the symposium.

Man & Woman, Boy & Girl had been in the making for the previous four years. Culling data from the hundreds of hermaphrodites who had passed through his Psychohormonal Research Unit since the early 1950s, and drawing (as Money announced in the book's preface) on scientific specialties as diverse as "genetics, embryology, neuroendocrinology, endocrinology, neurosurgery, social, medical and clinical psychology, and social anthropology," the book was a daunting, ambitious-looking effort of scholarship—all the more so for its often impenetrable Latinate terminology and convoluted syntactic structures. Its thematic thrust, however, was surprisingly straightforward and was reducible to one organizing idea stated again and again in its three hundred pages. It was the same idea Money had first advanced in his mid-1950s papers on intersexes: namely, that the primary factors driving human psychosexual differentiation are learning and environment, not biology.

Appearing five years after Money and Ehrhardt's data showing that female humans exposed to excesses of testosterone in utero displayed "tomboyism" in later life, *Man & Woman, Boy & Girl* had little choice but to acknowledge what Money called "a determining influence" of prenatal hormones on adult sexual behavior. Money explained that these influences were not decisive, however. Describing them as merely adding "a certain special flavor" to the girls' behavior, Money stated that in the formation of gender identity, prebirth biological influences are secondary to the power of postbirth environmental factors, which override them. To prove this nurturist bias, Money repeatedly evoked his principle of "matched pairs" of hermaphrodites—intersexual patients who shared a similar syndrome yet had been raised successfully, he claimed, as opposite sexes.

But the careful reader might have been struck by what looked like an uncharacteristic admission that hermaphrodites could not tell the whole story of human sexual development. For midway through the book, Money confessed to the frustrating constraints that prevented sex researchers from conducting the kinds of experiments that would provide truly conclusive answers to the riddle of psychosexual differentiation in humans. "The ultimate test of the thesis that gender identity differentiation is not preordained in toto by either the sex chromosomes, the prenatal hormonal pattern, or the postnatal hormonal levels would be undertaken, if one had the same ethical freedom of working in experiments with normal babies as with animals," he wrote. "Since planned experiments are ethically unthinkable, one can only take advantage of unplanned opportunities, such as when a normal boy baby loses his penis in a circumcision accident."

Then Money revealed that just such an "unplanned opportunity" to experiment on a developmentally normal infant had come his way—and that he had seized it. Describing how the injured baby's parents had allowed their son to be surgically reassigned as a girl, Money also pointed out what he called an "extreme unusualness" to the case: the child in question was one of a pair of identical male twins. The momentous import of this would not have been lost on either Money's readers or his AAAS audience. Money was saying that he had used for his experiment a pair of children whose biology was as close to identical as any two human beings could be: a pair of children whose lives had begun with the same primordial zygote cell, whose DNA bore the same genetic blueprint, and whose brains and nervous systems had developed in the womb within the same bath of prenatal hormones. In short, the ultimate matched pair.

That Money recognized the very special place Brenda Reimer's case occupied in his work—and indeed within the entire history of sex research—was clear from the emphasis he gave it in *Man & Woman, Boy & Girl*. First mentioned in the book's introduction, it was then cited at various key points throughout the text: in Chapter 8 on "Gender Identity Differentiation," in Chapter 9 on "Developmental Differentiation," in Chapter 10 on "Pubertal Hormones." It was in Chapter 7, on "Gender Dimorphism in Assignment and Rearing," that Money explored the case at greatest length, his account having been assembled from firsthand observation of Brenda during the family's annual visits to his Psychohormonal Research Unit and from letters and phone calls with Janet during the year.

Money made mention in passing of Brenda's "tomboyish traits" but dismissed these as insignificant next to the myriad ways she conformed to the stereotypes of female behavior—examples of which were selected from Janet's hopeful cataloging over the years of Brenda's fitful attempts to act more like a girl. Money did make reference to Brenda's extraordinary bathroom habits, but as he had done with Janet, he assured his readers that "many girls" attempt standing to urinate like boys, and he hinted that by age five Brenda no longer stood to pee—and that any sporadic reversion to her old habits was merely her effort at "copying her brother." No mention was made of the academic, social, and emotional difficulties that had obliged Money to intervene on Janet's behalf with the Winnipeg school authorities a year and a half before the book's publication.

By any measure, the account portrayed the experiment as an unqualified success. In comparison with her twin brother, Brenda provided what Money variously described as an "extraordinary" and a "remarkable" contrast. Brian's interest in "cars and gas pumps and tools" was compared with Brenda's avid interest in "dolls, a doll house and a doll carriage"; Brenda's cleanliness was characterized as wholly different from Brian's total disregard for such matters; Brenda's interest in kitchen work was placed alongside Brian's disdain for it. Money did describe Brenda as always the "dominant twin," though he gave the impression that this was changing over time. By age three, he reported, her dominance over Brian had become "that of a mother hen." All in all, the twins embodied an almost miraculous division of taste, temperament, and behavior along gender lines and seemed the "ultimate test" that boys and girls are made, not born.

The significance of the case was not lost on the then-burgeoning women's movement, which had been arguing against a biological basis for sex differences for decades. Money's own papers from the 1950s on the psychosexual neutrality of newborns had already been used as one of the main foundations of modern feminism. Kate Millet, in her bestselling 1970 feminist bible, *Sexual Politics*, had quoted the 1950s papers as scientific proof that the differences between men and women reflect not biological imperatives, but societal expectations and prejudices. The twins case offered still more dramatic, and apparently irrefutable, evidence to support that view.

"This dramatic case," *Time* magazine duly reported on January 8, 1973, the week after Money debuted the case at the AAAS meeting in Washington, "provides strong support for a major contention of women's liberationists: that conventional patterns of masculine and feminine behavior can be altered. It also casts doubt on the theory that major sexual differences, psychological as well as anatomical, are immutably set by the genes at conception."

The *New York Times Book Review* hailed *Man & Woman*,

Boy & Girl as "the most important volume in the social sciences to appear since the Kinsey reports." It summed up the book's argument on the power of nurture to override nature thus: "[I]f you tell a boy he is a girl, and raise him as one, he will want to do feminine things."

The twins case was quickly enshrined in myriad textbooks ranging from the social sciences to pediatric urology and endocrinology. "The clear message here is that even if biologically based sex differences in behavioral predispositions exist, social factors such as the sex which the child is assigned and in which the child is reared can substantially override and obscure them," wrote Alice G. Sargent about the case in her 1977 women's studies text, *Beyond Sex Roles*. Sociologists were equally enthralled by the case and cited it as the premier example of society's power to mold the most fundamental building block of human identity. Typical was the textbook *Sociology,* first published in 1977, in which Ian Robertson wrote that Money's work "indicates that children can easily be raised as a member of the opposite sex" and that what few inborn sex differences might exist in humans "are not clear-cut and can be overridden by cultural learning." The 1979 volume *Textbook of Sexual Medicine*, by Robert Kolodny and renowned sex researchers Masters and Johnson, cited the case as compelling evidence of the power of nurture over nature: "The childhood development of this (genetically male) girl has been remarkably feminine and is very different from the behavior exhibited by her identical twin brother. The normality of her development can be viewed as a substantial indication of the plasticity of human gender identity and the relative importance of social learning and conditioning in this process."

Money meanwhile did his part to ensure that the case got maximum exposure in both the academic and lay press.

Through the 1970s he made the case the centerpiece of his public addresses, rarely giving a speech in which he did not mention it. He soon introduced refinements into his crowd-pleasing presentation. At a March 1973 address at the prestigious Nebraska Symposium on Motivation, Money included a slide show in which he displayed a close-up photograph of Bruce's groin following the loss of his penis and a shot of the twins standing near a doorway. Brian is dressed in a short-sleeved shirt and dark trousers, Brenda in a sleeveless dress, white ankle socks, and white shoes. Money also showed a shot of Brenda alone, taken by Money himself. The child is seated awkwardly on the patterned upholstery of his office sofa. She wears a floral dress and running shoes, her bare left knee lifted self-protectively against the lens, her left hand deliberately obscuring her face. "In the last illustration," Money told his audience, "you have a pretty persuasive example of feminine body talk."

At his Nebraska lecture, Money also dropped a telling comment in summing up the case, when he told his listeners that Brenda's successful sex change refuted charges that "Money studies only odd and atypical cases, not normal ones." To those in the know, this was a not very veiled allusion to Money's principal theoretical rival, Milton Diamond.

In fact, Diamond did not object to Money's use of "odd and atypical cases" to study gender identity formation. He merely questioned the theoretical conclusions that Money drew from them. Since publishing his challenge to Money in 1965, Diamond had taken a teaching post at the University of Louisville in Kentucky, where he set to work studying intersexes himself. In his own interviews with intersexual patients, whom he met at the Louisville Children's Hospital, Diamond found that an imposed sex assignment in early infancy was by no means the magical panacea Money's writings suggested.

Instead, Diamond met several patients who contradicted the claim that rearing in a particular sex will always make a child accept that designation. There was the female baby exposed to excessive testosterone in utero, who was reared from birth as a girl but at age six stated to her mother that she was "a boy." There was the genetic male born with a tiny penis and raised as a girl, who at age seventeen voluntarily came to Louisville Children's Hospital requesting a change of sex to male—and was willing to endure more than twenty-five surgeries to construct an artificial penis, so vehemently was "she" determined to live in the sex of her genes and chromosomes. Even in those instances when an intersexual child *did* seem to accept a sex in contradiction to his or her biology, Diamond was not convinced that they had undergone a transformation in their core sexual identity. Such cases "should be considered a credit to human role flexibility and adaptability rather than an indelible feature of upbringing," he warned in the book *Perspectives in Reproduction and Sexual Behavior*, published in 1968.

In the years following publication of that book, Diamond was heartened to see that his views were beginning to be noticed by a scattering of scientists, researchers, and clinicians. In England, a pair of physicians, Dewhurst and Gordon, who had been treating intersexual patients for a decade, published their book, *The Intersexual Disorders*, in which they specifically questioned Money's assertion that rearing in a particular sex invariably led to a child's identifying with that sex. They not only cited a nationwide survey of British physicians whose clinical experience with intersexes contradicted Money's claim, but also referred to Diamond's work with intersexes in Louisville. A year later, in 1970, a fellow American joined Diamond for the first time in challenging Money's theory of human psychosexual differentiation.

Dr. Bernard Zuger was a Manhattan-based child psychiatrist whose work treating young male homosexuals and their families had caused him to question the prevailing view that sexual orientation results from rearing and environment. By exploring the family dynamics of his gay patients, Zuger discovered that in many cases the stereotypical pattern of an overbearing mother and a detached, hostile father did pertain; but by actually observing children in their family settings, Zuger came to believe that such a dynamic was not a *cause* of the child's homosexuality, but an *effect*. Long-term interviews with some fifty-five children (some of whom Zuger would follow for thirty years) showed that in virtually every case the boys demonstrated very early feminine play preferences, interests, and behavior. The father's efforts to bond over masculine interests were rebuffed by the child, and the father—rejected—would emotionally withdraw; the mother would move in to fill the vacuum, thus creating the observed pattern of a distant father and overbearing mother. Zuger suspected a biological basis for homosexuality that contradicted the universally accepted nurturist view—a view, as Zuger later wrote, that was founded to a remarkable degree on Money and the Hampsons' prize-winning 1950s papers on hermaphrodites. It was in an effort to learn how the Johns Hopkins team had arrived at those findings that Zuger submitted their work to close review.

Like the Canadian team more than a decade earlier, Zuger found serious problems with the Johns Hopkins team's methodology, interpretation of the clinical data, and statistical analysis. Noting that the papers were "lacking in such data as the ages when individual cases were observed, their subsequent course, and the part substitution therapy played in maintaining their gender role," Zuger also referred to new biological evidence, which had arisen in the intervening fifteen years, that cast further doubt on the Hopkins team's conclusions. Unlike the Canadian team, however, Zuger actually reanalyzed the

Johns Hopkins data using what he considered proper statistical methods and in light of the new biological findings. In doing so, he meticulously dismantled case after case cited by Money and the Hampsons and showed how children who, according to the team, had been raised in contradiction to their prevailing biological sex had in fact accepted a gender assignment in keeping with one or another of the factors that constitute a person's biological makeup as male or female: the chromosomes, the gonads, or the hormones. Summing up, Zuger wrote that of the sixty-five instances given as evidence for the dominance of rearing over biology, only four cases could be said to have escaped challenge—and even those were questionable. "The four cases," Zuger wrote, "might be explained on the basis of the 'flexibility' which Diamond attributes to human sexuality, or perhaps even by specific biologic factors which more detailed studies might have brought to light."

Slated for publication in a 1970 issue of the journal *Psychosomatic Medicine,* a prepublication copy of Zuger's paper was shown by the journal's editors to Money, who fired off a blistering response.

"It is difficult for the seeing to give art instruction to the blind," Money began, before proceeding to accuse Zuger of "intentionally biased sampling" and lambasting his work as "argumentative," and "very conjectural." Declining to address any of the specific scientific, methodological, and statistical unorthodoxies Zuger had highlighted, Money instead issued a threat to the journal editors: "I am sure you have ascertained, by now, the strength of my feeling about Dr. Zuger's manuscript. I do not want to take the easy way out and recommend simply that you do not publish it, because I know it would be equally easy, these days, to journal-shop and get the manuscript into print in another journal. What I really want is to ask Dr. Zuger to subject his manuscript to a very radical, total revision." A revision, in Money's exhaustive spelling out, that would bring Zuger's conclusions into agreement with Money's.

It was a measure of Money's academic power that the editors took his advice. They asked Zuger to revise his paper along the lines suggested by Money. Zuger declined, pointing out that Money had made no criticism "carrying any substance whatever" and adding, "Dr. Money's notion of a total revision, way beyond the scope of the paper, amounts to, of course, stalling it forever." Instead, through an arrangement agreed upon by both researchers, Zuger's paper and Money's letter of rebuttal were published in their entirety in the September-October 1970 edition of the journal.

Whatever larger debate might have been stimulated by the cumulative weight of the critiques by the Canadians in 1959, Diamond in 1965 and 1968, the British team in 1969, and Zuger in 1970 was effectively quashed by the fanfare that attended the publication, in late 1972, of Money's magnum opus, *Man & Woman, Boy & Girl*, and in particular its remarkable chapter on the twins case.

Dr. Mel Grumbach, a pediatric endocrinologist at the University of California, San Francisco, and a world authority on the subject, says that Money's twins case was decisive in the universal acceptance not only of the theory that human beings are psychosexually malleable at birth, but also of sex reassignment surgery as treatment of infants with ambiguous or injured genitalia. Once confined principally to Johns Hopkins, the procedure soon spread and today is performed in virtually every major country with the possible exception of China. While no annual tally of infant sex reassignments has ever been made, one physician conservatively estimates that three to five cases of babies with incongruous genitalia requiring sex change crop up annually in every major American city—giving the United States alone a total of at least one hundred such operations a year. Globally that figure could be as high as a thousand a year.

"Doctors were very influenced by the twin experience," Grumbach explains. "John stood up at a conference and said, 'I've got these two twins, and one of them is now a girl, and the other is a boy.' They were saying they took this normal boy and changed him over to a girl. That's powerful. That's *really* powerful. I mean, what is your response to that? This case was used to reinforce the fact that you can really do *anything*. You can take a normal XY male and convert it into a female in the neonatal period, and it won't make any difference." Grumbach adds, "John Money is a major figure, and what he says gets handed down and accepted as gospel by some."

But not all. Mickey Diamond had continued his research into how the sexual nervous system is organized before birth, and his studies had only strengthened his conviction that neither intersexual nor normal children were born psychosexually neutral—a conviction that would make him view with alarm the burgeoning practice of infant sex reassignment. And he was more convinced than ever that converting a normal infant from one sex to the other would be impossible. "But I didn't have any evidence to disprove the twins case at the time," Diamond says. "I didn't have anything except a theoretical argument to challenge it." He vowed to follow the case closely—a decision, he says, that was made from purely scientific motives. If, however, Diamond also by now felt a degree of personal involvement in his theoretical dispute with Money, that was perhaps understandable. For in the chapter directly following his account of the twins case in *Man & Woman, Boy & Girl*, Money had lashed out at Diamond and the others who had challenged his classic papers. Restating his own position,

Money had acidly observed: "It would not have been necessary to belabor this point, except that some writers still don't understand it," and he went on to say that the work of Diamond and the others was "instrumental in wrecking the lives of unknown numbers of hermaphroditic youngsters."

At the time of *Man & Woman, Boy & Girl*'s publication, Money and Diamond had limited their debate solely to published papers and books. That was shortly to change.

In September 1973, some nine months after the book's publication, John Money chaired the Third Annual International Symposium on Gender Identity, held at the Hotel Libertas in Dubrovnik, Yugoslavia. The symposium brought together a number of the leading authorities in the field of sexual development. These included Money's coauthor Dr. Anke Ehrhardt, who had taken a position as clinical associate professor in psychiatry at the State University of New York at Buffalo; Dr. Donald Laub, the Stanford Medical School professor and plastic surgeon who specialized in sex change surgery; and Dr. Ira Pauly, a psychiatrist who today is still a leader in the field of transexualism. Milton Diamond, not invited as either presenter or panelist, had nevertheless come to Yugoslavia to attend the conference. After the first day of speeches, during which Money had given the keynote address, the scientists gathered at an evening cocktail reception. The convivial gathering took place in a large room with vast windows that framed a view of the sunset over the Aegean Sea.

"I was sitting with some people over at one end of the room," Diamond recalls, "and Money was sitting over in another part of the room with Anke Ehrhardt. And all of a sudden he gets up and shouts at the top of his voice, 'Mickey Diamond, I hate your fucking guts!' "

An altercation ensued.

"They were arguing over the twins case," says Vern Bullough, then a professor at the State University of New York at Buffalo, and a friend of both men. "Mickey pointed out to John that all the data was not there, that it was too early to draw definitive conclusions about the kid. John suddenly slugged Mickey. Hit him. Mickey did not fight back. He just repeated, 'The data is not there.' John yelled at him, 'We have to stick together as sex researchers and not challenge one another!'" (Diamond says that he cannot recall any physical contact during this encounter.)

The combatants were separated, but the incident, Bullough says, threw a considerable pall over the party. Still, it did not inhibit Money's ongoing promotion of the twins case in lectures, published papers, and the press. The following June, Baltimore's *News American* newspaper ran a long profile on Money, in which the twins case was highlighted as his most impressive accomplishment in sex and gender research. "There isn't any question which one is the boy and which one the girl," Money told the newspaper. "It's just plain obvious."

"Such findings," the story continued, "could have an effect on future attitudes about sex roles that could prove comparable to that of Darwin's theory of Evolution."

5

≡

IN 1967, AT THE TIME of Brenda's castration, Dr. Money had stipulated to the Reimers that he see the child once a year for follow-up consultations. The trips, which were sometimes separated by as many as eighteen months, were meant to "guard against the psychological hazards" associated with growing up as a sex-reassigned child, as Money said in a letter to the Reimers' lawyer. According to the Reimers, however, and to contemporaneous clinical notes, the family's trips to the Psychohormonal Research Unit only exacerbated the confusion and fear that Brenda was already suffering. As Money's private case files show, Brenda reacted with terror on her first follow-up trip to Johns Hopkins at age four. "[T]here was something almost maniacal about her refusals [to be tested]," Money wrote in his notes, "and the way she hit, kicked and otherwise attacked people."

"You get the idea *something* happened to you," David says, explaining the dread that engulfed him during those mysterious annual visits to the Psychohormonal Research Unit, "but you don't know what—and you don't want to know." Brian, who was also required to submit to sessions with Dr. Money on each visit, found the trips equally bewildering and unsettling. "For the life of me I couldn't understand why, out of all the kids in my class, I'm the only one going with my sister to Baltimore to talk to this Dr. Money? It made us feel like we were aliens." The twins soon developed a conviction that everyone, from their parents to Dr. Money and his colleagues, was keeping something from them. "There was something not adding up," Brian says. "We knew that at a very early age. But we didn't make the connection. We didn't know."

All they did know was that Dr. Money and his associates seemed to take an inordinate amount of interest in everything about them. Some of the questions they were asked were relatively innocuous—"What's your favorite food?" "Who do you like more, Mom or Dad?" Others were less so. Dr. Money repeatedly asked the children about the differences between boys' and girls' genitalia and about what they knew about how babies were made. For Brenda, there were also private sessions with Dr. Money in which she was asked minutely detailed, numbingly repetitious questions about the toys she liked to play with, whether she fought with boys, whether she liked to play with girls. David says that Dr. Money and his coworkers dismissed Brenda's concerns about her boyish behavior and feelings. "They'd tell me, 'You shouldn't be *ashamed* of being a girl,'" David says. "They'd say, 'Girls can do the same things as boys.' One woman—an associate of Dr. Money's—told me, 'That's a typical tomboy thing; I did the same thing. You're just a tomboy.' But I was saying to myself, No, it's not *quite* like that. I don't think that's *quite* it."

Money's Psychohormonal Research Unit files corroborate

David's claim that Money and his colleagues seemed unwilling or unable to see and hear Brenda's efforts to tell them of her sexual confusion. At her earliest visits to the unit, Brenda could not consciously articulate her feelings of not being a girl, but as Money's notes show, those feelings were clear in her interviews and in the psychological tests Money and his students administered to her.

On a 19 June 1972 visit to the Psychohormonal Research Unit, when Brenda was six, she was given the Draw a Person Test, a standard test in which children demonstrate the primacy of their own gender identity by representing their own sex when instructed to draw a person. But Brenda did not draw a girl. Instead she produced the standard childish representation of a boy, which her tester, Money's student R. Clopper, called a "stick figure." Asked who it was, Brenda said, "Me." Asked to draw a figure of the sex *opposite* to herself, Brenda refused. Only after what the notes describe as "considerable coaxing" did she draw another stick figure, which she called "Brenda with a ponytail." Then she changed her response to "Brian," then changed again and said it was Brenda herself. Asked what the "opposite sex" figure to herself was wearing, Brenda said, "A dress."

David says he quickly learned to try to tell Money and his coworkers what they wanted to hear. And indeed, in Money's notes Brenda can sporadically be seen making sober avowals to her love of "sewing, cleaning, dusting and doing dishes." As Money's notes also show, however, Brenda often slipped up in her pose of serene and dutiful femininity. In one instance during the June 1972 visit, she can be seen actually feeling out Money for the correct way to answer him, and readjusting her response—on the fly—to fit her questioner's expectations.

The exchange began when Money asked if Brenda fought

back or ran away when boys started to fight her. Brenda at first blurted out, "Fight back," but then immediately reversed herself. "No," she said. "I just run away." Money, clearly noting this transparent attempt to tell him what he wanted to hear, asked the question again. Now Brenda could not be budged. She insisted that she did not fight boys—"Because I'm a girl."

"You're a girl?" the psychologist asked.

"And not a boy," Brenda felt compelled to assure him. Then, apparently unsure whether she had given the correct answer, she asked, "Girls don't fight, do they?"

Minutes later, when Money asked the question from yet another angle (Did she use her hands to fight people?), Brenda promptly contradicted her earlier avowals with the exclamation that she hit hard—"with my *fist*."

By the following year, when Brenda was seven, Money's notes show that she was less prone to such childish mistakes of inconsistency. When Money conducted his standard "schedule of inquiry" with her, she dutifully snapped out her answers with the swiftness of a call-and-response routine.

"Do you like to play house sometimes?" Money asked.

"Yes."

"Who plays mother?"

"Me."

"And who plays father?"

"My brother."

"And who is the baby?"

"My doll."

"How do you play with the dolls?"

"Feed them and, uh, give them milk. That's all."

At this same visit, however, Brenda's subconscious conviction that she was a boy emerged. For it was after the above exchange that Money asked Brenda to describe a "good dream." She began by describing a child on a farm with a horse. Before announcing the sex of the child, Brenda (as Money dictated in his notes) "paus[ed], and search[ed] for the next word" before revealing that the child was a boy.

"It was nice," Brenda continued, "and he wanted to eat, and he wanted to drink. He wanted to go to bed, and he wanted to sleep. That's all."

The presence of Brian in joint interviews with his sister did little to soften the impression Brenda gave of a scrappy, headstrong, dominant little pugilist. Indeed, Money's transcripts of his joint interviews with the twins only serve to reinforce an impression that family members, teachers, Child Guidance Clinic personnel, and others in Winnipeg described to me: that Brenda was the more traditionally masculine of the two children. When Money questioned the six-year-old twins about how to play with a doll, it was Brian who first spoke up, talking excitedly of how you hold, feed, and nurse them. Only when Brenda was pressed to respond did she try to parrot her brother's answer.

In this same interview, Money asked a question he would put to the twins repeatedly over the years: who was "the boss." Brian at first claimed that he was, but Money was clearly dubious. (Two years earlier, he had already noted that Brian "does a lot of copying of her.") He now repeated his question to Brian, asking if he truly was the boss. Brian's bravado instantly collapsed.

"I don't know," he admitted.

Brenda pounced. "*Are* you the boss?" she challenged him. "Do you *want* to be the boss? I don't think so. OK, *I'll* be the boss."

In this same joint interview, Money questioned the twins

about their respective fighting habits. Brian said he fought—
but only with girls, and in particular a little girl with orange
hair who picked on him.

"Do you fight with other boys?" Money asked.

"No," Brian said. "I fight with girls." Brenda then
explained that she defended Brian against his female antago-
nists, telling them, "You better not hit my brother."

Brenda was still more explicit about her role as Brian's
protector a year later. In an interview alone with Money, she
once again described how she rescued Brian from bullies. At
the same time she let slip that she sometimes bullied Brian
herself.

"Do you and Brian fight sometimes?" Money asked.

"Yep," Brenda said.

"Do you fight with your hands, or fists, or feet—or how?"

"Fists and feet and hands."

"Can you beat Brian up, or does he beat you?"

"I could beat him up."

"Who wins?"

"I do."

It was at this same visit that Money compared how the
twins threw a ball. Brian had privately told the psychologist
that Brenda threw "like a girl." To test this exciting thesis,
Money gave Brenda a ball of modeling clay and asked her to
throw it. "[S]he pitched the ball in a fairly straightforward
way from her left hand (both children are left handed),"
Money dictated in his private notes. "It was a standard over-
hand throw."

David says that at seven he was still too young to be able to
formulate in words his inner sense of being identical to his
brother in every way but in the anatomy of his genitals. Brenda,
though, can be seen clearly struggling to articulate this concept
in an exchange with Money over the difference between boys'

and girls' private parts. It was a topic that Money had quizzed the twins on since their earliest visits to the unit and one that clearly caused both children acute embarrassment. In the present instance, Brenda dodged and weaved for several minutes, too mortified and frightened to say the words *penis* and *vagina*. Instead she employed a number of stalling tactics that she had perfected over the years in her verbal dueling matches with Money. To his question about how to tell boys and girls apart, she first offered that a boy has short hair, a girl long. Money asked the question again. Brenda said that boys wear pants, girls dresses. This went on for several more minutes until Money, clearly growing impatient, said, "Well, I'll help you. You have a look down here, between the legs. How is a boy and how is a girl down there? What's the difference?"

"You mean it's flat?" Brenda said.

"A boy has a penis—for peeing through," Money said. "It is just like a little sausage, huh? What does a girl have?"

"I don't know."

"Well, she has it flat," Money said. He continued: "A boy doesn't have that. They are both different." Money repeated: "They are both different. Now we know, don't we?"

At this point Money's private notes continue: "Spontaneously she adds: 'But we're twins. We're twins.' "

Money, obviously taken aback by the vehemence of this rare outburst from the ordinarily tight-lipped girl, asked, "What does it mean when you say you're twins?"

Brenda helplessly cataloged several of the physical things that made her identical to her brother: their left-handedness, their voices, their eyes. Too ashamed to speak directly of her genitals, she left it up to Money to settle the mystery of how two such completely similar children could be "both different" in their anatomic sex. But Money failed, or declined, to catch Brenda's meaning, and instead returned to his standard schedule of inquiry—the list of prepared questions about toys, friends, school, and fighting that he worked through at each visit.

As the twins got older, Money's questioning grew more explicit. "Dr. Money would ask, 'Do you ever dream of having sex with women?'" Brian says. "'Do you ever get an erection?' And the same with Brenda. 'Do you think about this? About that?'"

While attempting to probe the twins' sexual psyches, Money also tried his hand at programming Brenda's and Brian's respective sense of themselves as girl and boy. One of his theories of how children form their different *gender schemas*—Money's term—was that they must understand at a very early age the differences between male and female sex organs. Pornography, he believed, was ideal for this purpose. "[E]xplicit sexual pictures," he wrote in his book *Sexual Signatures,* "can and should be used as part of a child's sex education." Such pictures, he said, "reinforce his or her own gender identity/role."

"He would show us pictures of kids—boys and girls— with no clothes on," Brian says. David recalls that Dr. Money also showed them pictures of adults engaged in sexual intercourse. "He'd say to us, 'I want to show you pictures of things that moms and dads do.'"

Money had two sides to his personality, according to the twins: "One when Mom and Dad weren't around," Brian says, "and another when they were." When their parents were present, Money was avuncular, mild-mannered. Alone with the children he could be irritable or worse, especially when they defied him. They were particularly resistant, the twins say, to Money's requests that they remove their clothes and inspect each other's genitals. David recalls an occasion when he attempted to defy the psychologist. "He told me to take my clothes off," David says, "and I just did not do it. I just stood there. And he screamed, '*Now!*' Louder than that. I thought he was going to give me a whupping. So I took my clothes off and stood there, shaking." In a separate conversation with me, Brian recalls that same incident. "'Take your clothes off—*now!*'" Brian shouts.

Though the children could not know this, the genital inspections that Dr. Money demanded they perform were central to his theory of how children develop a sense of themselves as boy or girl—and thus, in Money's mind, crucial to the successful outcome of Brenda's sex reassignment. For as Money stressed in his writings of the period, "The firmest possible foundations for gender schemas are the differences between male and female genitals and reproductive behavior, a foundation our culture strives mightily to withhold from children. All young primates explore their own and each others' genitals, masturbate, and play at thrusting movements and copulation—and that includes human children everywhere, as well as subhuman primates. The only thing wrong about these activities is not to enjoy them."

But the children did not enjoy these enforced activities—particularly those involving "play at thrusting movements and copulation," which Brian recalls that Dr. Money first introduced when the twins were six years old. Money, he says, would make Brenda assume a position on all fours on his office sofa and make Brian come up behind her on his knees and place his crotch against her buttocks. Variations on the therapy included Brenda lying on her back with her legs spread and Brian lying on top of her. On at least one occasion, Brian says, Dr. Money took a Polaroid photograph of them while they were engaged in this part of the therapy.

Of all the therapy the children received, this particular

form of counseling left the deepest impression on both twins. Today David is still unwilling to speak about it. "There are some things I don't *want* to remember," he says. In 1989 he did describe the sessions to Jane Fontane, the woman who would become his wife. The two had just watched a TV documentary on CIA torture involving electroshock to people's genitals. "He cried hysterically," Jane told me. "He was crying about John Money. I'd never seen him like that. I tried to comfort him. David said Dr. Money made him go on all fours and made Brian go up behind his butt. They were being photographed. He mentioned that very act."

Brian speaks of the coital mimicry only with the greatest emotional turmoil. "It's very hard to— I don't understand why to this day we were forced to do that," Brian says.

Brian's perplexity would have instantly been eradicated had he ever made a study of John Money's theory of childhood sexual rehearsal play, articulated repeatedly in books, papers, speeches, and press interviews published over a quarter century, and its supposed critical importance in the establishment of healthy gender identity.

Money's fascination with the topic of coital mimicry in children had its origins in a trip he made in late 1969 to the northern coast of Australia with three professors from the University of New South Wales. There Money visited for two weeks in a village of coastal aborigines called the Yolngu—a tribe Money would later describe as wholly heterosexual and entirely free of any psychosexual gender confusions or dysfunction whatsoever. While visiting one of the tribal elementary schools, Money heard a secondhand report from an eight-year-old child "that two six-year-old relatives at the camp-fire the previous night had given a demonstration of nigi-nigi"—a term Money understood to mean, through his preteen interpreter, "sexual intercourse." This incident, coupled with Money's belief in the tribe's lack of any gender confusion, was the foundation for his theory that childhood "sexual rehearsal play" was vital to the formation of a healthy adult gender identity—a theory he first articulated in a 1970 paper on the Yolngu published in the *British Journal of Medical Psychology.*

"The straightforward attitude of the Yolngu towards nudity and sex play in young children allows these children to grow up with a straightforward attitude towards sex differences, towards the proper meaning and eventual significance of the sex organs, and towards their own reproductive destiny and sense of identity as male or female," he wrote. Conversely, Money hypothesized, Western society's restrictions on such sex play in young children was highly detrimental and was the root cause of such things as homosexuality, pedophilia, and lust murders.

One of Money's colleagues on the trip, Professor J. E. Cawte, who has studied the Yolngu for almost thirty years, says that he has never witnessed sexual rehearsal play among the tribal children and knows of no researcher who has. Professor Cawte is similarly mystified at the claim that adults of the Yolngu manifest no sexual difficulties. As a psychiatrist who has ministered to the needs of the tribe for decades, Cawte says he has treated many of the Yolngu adults for a wide variety of what he calls "sexual neuroses" and dysfunctions of every variety.

Nevertheless, the Yolngu's purported habit of childhood sexual rehearsal play and their alleged freedom from any psychosexual confusion became a constant reference in almost every public utterance of Money's for the next three decades. He included a section on sexual rehearsal play in *Man & Woman, Boy & Girl* and published an article on the theory in *The Sciences* magazine in 1975. By the time he came to write

Sexual Signatures in the mid-1970s (a time concurrent with his treatment of the Reimer twins), the issue of childhood sexual rehearsal play had assumed the dimensions of a crusade—and one that could move Money to shrill flights of rhetoric. "[W]hat happens in our culture?" he wrote. "Children's sex explorations are treated like a contagious disease. . . . [D]on't let them see the incontrovertible differences in their genitals, and don't, at all costs, let them rehearse copulation—the one universal human activity that still imperatively demands that the two sexes behave differently and harmoniously!"

In an interview with the pornographic magazine *Genesis* in April 1977, Money vented his frustration against the prohibition against childhood sexual rehearsal play and a psychologist's right to observe it. "The number of studies of the effects of depriving human infants and juveniles of sexual rehearsal play is exactly and precisely zero," he said, "because anyone who tried to conduct such a study would risk imprisonment for contributing to the delinquency of minors, or for being obscene. Just imagine the headlines and the fate of a research-grant application requesting funds to watch children playing fucking games!" He sounded the same theme in a 1984 speech, lamenting that it was a "crime" for a sexologist "to make a pictorial record of children's normal, healthy sexual rehearsal play" and returned to this theme in *Psychology Today* when he showed a book with pictures of young children engaged in sexual intercourse to interviewer Constance Holden and said, "You have just become a criminal by looking at those pictures of children."

In a 1988 appearance on *The Oprah Winfrey Show*, Money unexpectedly veered from the show's main topic (intersexuality) and put in a plug for his pet theory. "I worked among the aboriginal people on the north coast of Australia in the early seventies," Money told Oprah's audience. "I was very interested in the fact that they don't impose a sexual taboo on themselves, and they don't punish children for doing normal sexual rehearsal play . . . and I was very surprised to find out that there were no bisexual or no gay people in there." Oprah, who had clearly not been briefed on this particular aspect of Money's research, tried to deflect the remark. "I'm almost afraid to ask what all that means, Dr. Money," she interjected. Money, however, was not to be put off, and continued with an explicit description of the sexual rehearsal play he now claimed to have directly witnessed among the Yolngu. A year later, Money could still be heard trying to promote his theory on an episode of the Canadian TV show *The Originals,* where he scoffingly referred to the prudery of a society that prohibits such childhood exploration. "It has become very obvious to me," he said, "that sexual rehearsal play is part of nature's absolute intention, in order to allow children to grow up to be sexually normal."

But never having heard of Money's theory of sexual rehearsal play, Brian and Brenda Reimer could only perform the ritualized poses obediently, in complete perplexity about their meaning and wholly unaware of the critical role their counselor understood the episodes to have in the successful outcome of his most famous experiment in infant sex change.

Not surprisingly perhaps, Brenda, at age seven, began strongly to resist going to Baltimore. Money suggested to Ron and Janet that they sweeten the pill of the annual visits by blending the trips to Johns Hopkins with a family vacation. "Soon," Janet says, "we were promising Disneyland and side trips to New York just to get her to go."

It was also at this time that Dr. Money began increasingly to focus on the issue of vaginal surgery in his sessions with

Brenda. When she underwent her castration at the age of twenty-two months, Brenda was only at the first stage of the feminizing process. Dr. Jones had elected to wait until Brenda's body was closer to fully grown before performing the two remaining surgeries: the first to lower her urethra into the female position, the second to excavate a full vaginal canal. For Dr. Money, there was an increasingly urgent need for Brenda to prepare for these operations. Because genital appearance was critical to his theory of how one "learns" a sexual identity, he believed that Brenda's psychological sex change could not be complete until her physical sex change was finished.

There was only one problem. Brenda was determined not to have the surgery—ever. As Money's private clinical notes reveal, he first raised the issue of vaginal surgery with Brenda on her visit of 24 April 1973. He segued into the subject with deceptive casualness.

"That reminds me of something else I wanted to tell you about," Money said after interrogating her at length on the usual range of topics: fighting, how to tell boys and girls apart. "You know already the way you are made down there, between your legs, you are not exactly the same as other girls, eh?"

"Yes," Brenda said. She was understating the case considerably. Her vagina, with its small stumplike protrusion under the skin and its apparent scarring, caused her such confusion and anxiety that she could not even bring herself to look, or touch, between her own legs.

"Well, I have a message for you about that," Money said. "Here in this hospital we can fix it up for you and make it look like it's supposed to look."

"Huh?" Brenda said.

Money went on to explain that the doctors could operate on her so that she could urinate properly. (It was Money's theory that Brenda's continuing unorthodoxies in the bath-room resulted solely from the condition of her uncompleted vaginal surgery.) "How old will you be when you're ready for that [operation]?" Money asked.

Brenda resorted to the reply she so often gave to Money's queries. "I don't know."

Money suggested that Brenda would be ready at her next visit, when she was eight—one year away. Brenda said nothing. Money talked on at length about the "doctor in the white coat" who would "fix it up down there." Finally Brenda found her voice.

"I wouldn't do that," she said.

This was a position from which Brenda would refuse to shift.

Today David explains that his refusal to undergo vaginal surgery was not only a result of his deep fear of hospitals, doc-tors, and needles. It had to do with certain realizations he came to around this time—realizations that convinced him he was not a girl and never would be, no matter what his parents, his doctor, his teachers, or anyone else said. For as David explains, when seven-year-old Brenda daydreamed of an ideal future, she saw herself as a twenty-one-year-old male with a mustache, a sports car, and surrounded by admiring friends. "He was some-body I wanted to *be*," David says today, reflecting on those childhood fantasies. Based on those fantasies, Brenda was con-vinced that to submit to vaginal surgery would lock her into a gender that was not her own.

Dr. Money, with the fate of his famous case hanging in the balance, spared no effort to break down the child's resis-tance. The transcript of their encounter on 24 April 1973 continues with Money taking a new tack. Hoping to teach Brenda about the vaginal opening and canal, which she did not yet possess, Money asked, "How much do you know about where babies come from?"

Brenda said, "From their mother's tummy."

"Now," Money said, circling closer to the issue at hand, "do you know how the baby gets out?"

Brenda, clearly tumbling to Money's tactic, stalled, mumbling incoherent syllables.

"When it's ready to get born," Money repeated, "how does it get out?"

Again Brenda stalled.

"I'll ask my question one more time," Money said. "When the baby is ready to get born, how does it get out from inside the mother? Where does it get out?"

Brenda, aware that she had driven Money to the limits of his patience, feigned not to have understood. "Oh!" she now exclaimed. "The mother gets her out."

Money was not to be put off so easily. "How does the mother get it out?" he repeated.

"Um, I don't know," Brenda finally said. "I didn't learn that at school."

"Would you like me to show you some pictures?" Money said.

Brenda made no recorded response.

"This is a book called *Two Births,*" Money continued, opening a large coffee-table book for Brenda to look at.

Published one year earlier, *Two Births* is a vintage artifact of the early 1970s. Photographed by Ed Buryn, it is a record of two hippie women having home births. The large black-and-white photographs are expertly and beautifully made but are at the same time unsparingly graphic in their depiction of the moments before, during, and after birth. Intense close-ups show both women naked, grimacing, their bare breasts swollen, their vaginas distended as the babies' heads begin to push through the stretched orifices.

"See, there is the lady with the baby inside," Money said

as he leafed through the pages for Brenda. "Getting ready, almost ready to come out. . . . See, here's the baby just getting ready to come out and here it's really coming out. See, there's his head beginning to poke through. . . . There, it got all the way out."

"Now," Money continued, "I wanted to show you that picture of a baby being born because I wanted to tell you that, down there, the way you are, you can't find the baby hole yet." And suddenly Money was once again talking about the "doctor in the hospital here" who could give her a "baby hole."

Neither the pictures of the grimacing women with the spread legs and stretched vaginas nor Money's explanations of the pictures convinced Brenda to submit to the vaginal surgery. Nor did what followed—a description from Dr. Money of sexual intercourse.

"A lot of kids don't know that story," Money said when he had finished describing how the penis goes into the vagina, "because they don't have a doctor to tell them. The lucky kids who know about it are best if they don't talk about it too much."

"Yes," Brenda said.

"You are pretty wise, aren't you?"

"No," Brenda said.

"I think so."

"No," Brenda said. "I'm not."

"Aren't you?" Money persisted.

Brenda did not reply.

"How are you?" Money asked.

Brenda said nothing.

"I think you're a wise girl," Money said.

"No," Brenda repeated, "I'm not."

"You're one of my favorite girls."

According to David, Money's supposed affection for
Brenda turned to increasing frustration, impatience, and
anger as she continued to resist his blandishments. Brenda
meanwhile reacted badly to the increasing pressure to submit
to the operation. In the spring of 1974, facing another summer visit to Dr. Money's Psychohormonal Research Unit and
yet another battle of wits and wills with him, Brenda found
that the pressure was simply too much.

"I had a nervous breakdown," David says. "Because I
knew, also, that right after I saw this guy on the summer hol-
idays it would be *school*. It was a double whammy. I remember the summer I turned nine just huddling in a corner and
shaking and crying."

Seeing their daughter's distress, Ron and Janet postponed
that summer's visit. Finally, however, it was Ron, convinced that
only Dr. Money could help their daughter, who insisted
that Brenda return to Johns Hopkins in the fall. And so on 19
November 1974 the family again visited the Psychohormonal
Research Unit. The two-day visit was a trial for all concerned—
but especially for Brenda. In a one-on-one taped interview,
Money tried in vain to get her to speak. She would only mum-
ble monosyllables. When Money tried to raise the topic of vaginal surgery, Brenda scurried from the room, found her father in
the hallway, and refused to leave his side.

Today David recognizes that if he had told his parents what
went on between Brenda and the psychologist behind closed
doors—the pressure tactics, cajoling, pornography, and un-
orthodox inspections and posings—Janet and Ron would never
have made her return to Johns Hopkins. But the thought never
occurred to her—for a simple and chilling reason.

"I thought my parents *knew*," David says. "I figured, they're
responsible for me. They brought me here. They *must* know
what's going on."

6

≡

Ron and Janet did not know what went on in the twins' sessions with Dr. Money. "The twins would be whisked off somewhere, I didn't know where," Janet says. "Dr. Money spent some of the time in a little office talking mostly with me, some to Ron." They had no reason to think that the psychologist was any different with Brenda and Brian than he was with them, and with Ron and Janet he was unfailingly polite and kind. Only once did they have any reason to suspect that there might be another side to Dr. Money. "One time we came into his office when he wasn't expecting us," Ron says, "and he was giving all holy shit to his secretary. Just *chewing* her out for something small—she forgot to mail a letter or something. When he saw us, he let it drop."

This unsettling glimpse was never repeated, so Ron and Janet wrote it off as a rare moment when the psychologist lost control. Otherwise they continued to think of Money as their closest confidant and friend. And he considered them important allies in his ongoing struggles with Brenda. In fact, the end of their fraught November 1974 visit, Dr. Money took Ron and Janet aside and gave them what he called a "homework assignment," telling them to find opportunities to talk with Brenda explicitly about her genitalia and vaginal surgery and impressing upon them how important it was that she agree, at the very next visit, to a vaginal inspection.

In a private note to himself after this meeting, Money was still more emphatic: "Next year it will be imperative for a physical examination to be done," he wrote. "There is an optimal length of time for dealing with a difficult issue by avoiding it, and that optimum will be passed next year, if it is not already passed this year." Something of Money's growing frustration with Brenda's stalwart resistance also crept into this note. "When Brenda is tense and hyperkinetic, she does not give an exactly endearing impression nor a particularly feminine one."

Back in Winnipeg, Ron and Janet got to work on their homework assignment. Told to impress upon Brenda the differences between male and female sex organs, Ron and Janet had been instructed by Money to allow her to see them naked. In *Sexual Signatures*, Money emphasized the importance of such parental genital displays for correct heterosexual child development, and even went so far as to recommend that parents engage in sexual intercourse in front of their children. "With a little calm guidance," he wrote, "the experience can be integrated into the child's sex education and serve to reinforce his or her own gender identity/role."

Janet and Ron drew the line at having sex in front of the twins, but Janet did try to follow the other parts of the homework assignment. She appeared naked, as often as possible, in front of Brenda. This only embarrassed the child, who seemed startled to see her mother walking around the house unclothed. "All of a sudden," David recalls, "right after we go on one of

John Money's trips, she's walking around stark naked." Desperate for the treatment to work, and afraid to contravene Money's orders in the least, Janet persevered. "He encouraged us to go to a nude beach," she says. "We knew of a river where there was nobody for miles around. Ron and I went in the buff, but the twins wouldn't." Janet also tried, in conversation, to "break the ice" with Brenda about the vaginal surgery, but with similar dismal results. "The minute I went anywhere near that topic," Janet says, "she'd leave the room."

The atmosphere in the Reimer home grew steadily more tense as Brenda realized that her parents were now working in collusion with Dr. Money to force her into the surgery. She began to rebel against her parents openly. Even the supposedly happy occasion of Christmas became an ordeal. Brenda raged against having to get into the party dress her parents insisted she wear when they went to see Ron's family in Kleefeld. Brenda had always hated going to see her extended family because this always meant that her parents would put special pressure on her to dress and act like a little lady. Making matters worse, her grandparents, aunts, and uncles would constantly scrutinize her. "They'd be studying me like a bug, to see how much I'd changed throughout the year," David says. "And as soon as I'd catch them staring at me, they'd look the other way. I told my dad, 'I don't know why, but I always feel like an oddball around my own family.' He said, very quietly, 'I know.'"

Ron's family, like the rest of the relatives, knew about Brenda's sex change, so Ron understood why they studied his daughter so closely. He also recognized in his heart of hearts what they were seeing. "*I* sort of knew it wasn't working after Brenda was seven or something," Ron says. "But what were we going to do?"

Neither Ron nor Janet could entertain the notion that they

had made the wrong decision. The only option was to put distance between themselves and anyone who seemed bent on making them face such a realization. From now on, Ron decided, they would see as little of his parents as possible.

But it proved difficult to segregate themselves from all reminders of Brenda's problems. Just that fall the Child Guidance Clinic had once again contacted them to say that her behavioral problems in school had worsened and that she was "hyper and defiant" and looked "unhappy." Furthermore, the clinic reported, Brian was also showing signs of increasingly serious emotional problems related to Brenda's predicament.

"At that point my main emotion toward my sister was jealousy," Brian explains. "She got all the attention. I was just the normal one. Mom and Dad were so worried about Brenda that they neglected me. I felt I was unimportant. I started to act up a bit, try to get some attention." He succeeded that March, when he was caught trying to shoplift from a local store and the proprietor threatened to press charges. For Janet and Ron, this proved to be the last straw.

At the time of Brenda's sex reassignment almost eight years earlier, their local pediatrician had advised them to move away from the area so that they could make a fresh start in a place where there was no lingering memory of their former son. They had refused his advice at the time. Now they saw the wisdom of it. It was imperative that they get away from the ghosts and doubters who haunted Winnipeg; it was imperative that they put as much distance as possible between themselves and Ron's parents, the Child Guidance Clinic—everyone.

That spring of 1975, Ron and Janet sold their house, their furniture, their appliances, and their '66 Pontiac. They bought a half-ton Chevy truck with a camper on the back. They packed up what few belongings they still owned and headed west for British Columbia. Ron had a friend out there who'd told him there was plenty of work. Yet so little had Ron planned this move—so completely had he failed to look ahead—that he would later castigate himself for having sold all their possessions and thus put himself in the position of having to buy everything when they got to BC.

"I remember thinking when we got there, Oh God, what did I *do*?" Ron says. "How could I have just picked up and moved? What an *idiot* thing to do!" Only much later, Janet says, did she and Ron fully face why they had so precipitately uprooted their lives and headed off to BC. "We were trying to escape."

That Dr. Money already understood this motive was clear from a note he made to himself at this time. "The plan to move to British Columbia may include a bit too much geographical magic," he wrote, "especially with regard to solving problems with the grandparental families. However, it could also turn out to be a perfectly satisfactory move."

Their destination was British Columbia's mountainous, wooded, sparsely populated interior. They settled in a tiny place called Ashton Creek. The nearest town was Enderby with a population of just 2,500. Ron bought a house trailer, which they parked in an encampment. The twins were enrolled in grade four at tiny Ashton Creek School.

"It was more of a country school," David says. "But it didn't matter what kind of school it was. If you're not comfortable, you're not going to be comfortable no matter what school you go to. You can go to a thousand schools, and it's always the same. Because the standard rule of thumb is: There's the girls over here, and there's the boys over there. Separated. Which direction [do I go]? There's no belonging. So you're an outcast. It doesn't change. School to school to school. It doesn't change."

In April the family returned to Baltimore for another visit with Dr. Money. By now, Brenda, almost ten years old, had developed a new attitude toward Dr. Money. Frowning, sullen, and almost completely mute, she refused to answer his questions in anything but grunting monosyllables. She also imagined that she had succeeded in keeping secret certain shameful impulses she had started to have, but she was wrong. According to Ron, it was during this visit that Dr. Money informed him of an issue that had arisen during his private sessions with Brenda.

"Money told us that he had asked Brenda what partner she would rather have, a boy or a girl," Ron recalls. "Brenda had said, 'A girl.' " Ron says that Dr. Money wanted to know how they felt about raising a lesbian. At a loss for how to respond, but relieved that Dr. Money did not seem to think it significant, Ron said what he honestly believed about homosexuality: "It's not the most important thing in life."

Money evidently agreed, for this clinical finding was not included in his next report on the twins, which appeared later that year in *Archives of Sexual Behavior*. Entitled "Ablatio Penis" (the Latin term for the medical condition of complete amputation of the organ), the paper recapped earlier data about the sex reassignment's success and added one new piece of evidence of the girl's happy femininity. Money recounted an exchange he had had with Brenda about the family's recent trip to the Washington Zoo: "I resorted to the standard question of which animal she'd want to be if she could change into one," Money reported. "She elected to be a monkey. . . . 'Would you want to be a boy monkey or a girl monkey?' I asked. 'A girl one,' she replied, and gave as the reason for this choice, 'I'm already a girl!' "

A question remains about this seemingly unequivocal statement of female gender identity (even if not dismissed as one of Brenda's typical efforts at telling the psychologist what he wanted to hear). In that interview session of 24 April 1973, Money had threaded his reel-to-reel tape recorder incorrectly. Thus Brenda's statements on the tape were virtually inaudible, and Money had to make a special effort to hear anything at all of the interview. "I'm pressing the earpiece closer into my ear," he dictated in his notes while listening to the playback of this exchange, "and hearing a little more now. . . . I ask her why she wants to be a monkey, but I cannot hear the reply on tape. I remember that it was something that I did not immediately understand until she demonstrated with her hands that she meant climbing and swinging. I then asked her if she would want to be a boy monkey or a girl monkey. Her reply is audible on tape, 'a girl one.' I inquire as to why. . . . Again, the reply is audible on the tape, 'I'm already a girl.' The pronunciation of *girl* is as if it were spelled g-r-i-r-l."

Upon seeing these interview transcripts for the first time, in 1998, David insists that he did not say "girl" but in fact used one of the standard evasion tactics he had by then developed. Instead of answering Money's question about the *sex* of the monkey, Brenda had instead answered what *kind* of monkey she would like to be. "I said 'gorilla,' " David says. Considering the particular clipped Canadian prairie accent in which all the Reimers speak, it is easy to see how the word *gorilla*, heard through a faulty recording, would come out "grirl." That it should then be interpreted by Money as "girl" is perhaps illustrative not of Brenda's gender identity but rather of the role the subjective hopes of scientific researchers can play in the gathering and interpretation of their data.

Epistemological vagaries notwithstanding, Money's "Ablatio Penis" paper ended on a note of high optimism. "No one [outside the family] knows [that she was born a boy]," Money wrote. "Nor would they ever conjecture. Her behavior is so normally that of an active little girl, and so clearly different by contrast from the boyish ways of her twin brother, that it offers nothing to stimulate anyone's conjectures."

Later that year, Money published yet another account of Brenda's successful metamorphosis. This time the intended audience was not only Money's scientific and medical colleagues, but the general public. The new account appeared in *Sexual Signatures*. Coauthored with journalist Patricia Tucker, the book was couched in the language of commercial poppsych bestsellers, and it represented Money's bid for a wider audience. It also provided his most detailed and readable account of Brenda's sex change to date. Stripped of the often impenetrable medical jargon that characterized his earlier accounts of the sex reassignment, *Sexual Signatures* offered an unrelievedly upbeat, almost triumphant version of Brenda's story.

"Although the girl had been the dominant twin in infancy," Money wrote, "by the time the children were four years old there was no mistaking which twin was the girl and which the boy. At five, the little girl already preferred dresses to pants, enjoyed wearing her hair ribbons, bracelets and frilly blouses, and loved being her daddy's little sweetheart. Throughout childhood, her stubbornness and the abundant physical energy she shares with her twin brother and expends freely have made her a tomboyish girl, but nonetheless a .girl." Describing Brenda's sex reassignment as "[d]ramatic proof that the gender identity option is open at birth for normal infants," Money went on to claim that the child's subsequent history was proof of how well the family had adjusted to the original decision in favor of castration.

Even as *Sexual Signatures* appeared in bookstores, the Reimer family's adjustment to their decision was growing more imperiled by the day in British Columbia.

Ron, who had found work in a sawmill after a grueling period of unemployment, was no better than he had ever been at talking about his daughter and the major medical decisions that were ahead of her. "I'm a workaholic," Ron admits. "If I'm worried about something, I just work harder." Rather than face what was happening with Brenda—her nervous breakdown before the previous year's trip to Johns Hopkins, her intense boyishness, her refusal to discuss the surgery, her continued dismal performance in school, her "lesbianism"—Ron would simply stagger home from an overtime shift at the sawmill, silently shovel in his dinner, then stare into the TV while he drained a six-pack. Often failing to join Janet in bed, he would simply slope off into unconsciousness in front of the TV.

Janet was faring little better. After six months in British Columbia she was feeling dangerously alienated. "I had no family to talk to," she says. "I had some friends, but they didn't know the real me—or the real Brenda." The only person who *did* know the real Brenda was Ron, and he refused to talk about her. David recalls vividly the chaos that engulfed their small trailer: "Mom crying and screaming," he says, "Dad drinking."

That summer Janet's condition deteriorated. She sank into a serious depression and found herself obsessively thinking about all that had happened to them. "Sometimes it didn't feel real," she says. "What I especially found difficult was all those years I had a strong sense of Christianity, of a living God—a God who laid out a path for you. I remember thinking, What kind of a purpose could this *possibly* have in life? All this pain after pain after pain? What possible purpose could there be in this *horrible* life?" She began to suffer wild mood swings, from volatile anger to weeping despondency. At times, she felt that her very sanity was in jeopardy. Janet says that she experienced periods of "psychosis"—episodes when she could not tell reality from fantasy.

"She was unpredictable," Brian says. "It was like walking on eggs. You didn't know what you were going to come home to." Janet consulted some doctors in the area. "I couldn't get help," she says. "One lady doctor said to me, 'Oh, all you need is another baby to keep you busy.' I said, 'The last thing I need is another child!' "

Ron and Janet were almost completely estranged. That summer Janet drifted into an affair with one of the local men to spite Ron. He found out and was devastated. Janet, guilt-ridden, swallowed a bottle of sleeping pills. Ron found her in time to drive her to the hospital in Enderby. Upon Janet's release, the couple talked about divorce but decided to soldier on somehow together. In the early fall, more bad luck arrived: their house trailer caught fire and burned to the ground, destroying all the family pictures and most of their possessions.

In November 1976, one year and five months after their flight from Winnipeg, the family packed up the few belongings that had escaped the fire and began the long drive back to Winnipeg. Janet and Ron were obliged to admit that their attempt to escape had only exacerbated the problems they were trying to flee. Janet's depression and suicide attempt, the near breakup of the marriage, and the acceleration in Ron's alcohol intake had all taken a visible toll on the twins. Brian was now beginning to have troubling outbursts of frustrated violence and anger against other kids. Brenda turned her feelings inward and became increasingly anxiety-ridden and depressed. She was also demonstrating overt hostility and distrust toward both parents, especially her mother— although, as David points out, he tried to hide these feelings because he was now trying with everything he had to hold together his parents' disintegrating marriage. "I thought it was all *my* fault," David explains. "So I would try to make them happy. I would try to be more ladylike."

Those efforts proved more difficult than ever for Brenda— especially now that she had passed her eleventh birthday, and certain physiological changes began to occur: her shoulders had started to widen and grow more muscular; her neck and biceps, too, began to thicken; and sometimes now her voice would crack into a strange squeaking sound.

All in all, the Reimers' sojourn in British Columbia formed a bitterly ironic contrast to the way their lives were portrayed in the *New York Times Book Review* of May 1975, when reviewer Linda Wolfe, working from the evidence presented by John Money in *Sexual Signatures*, wrote of "the identical twin boy whose penis was cauterized at birth and who, now that his parents have opted for surgical reconstruction to make him appear female, has been sailing contentedly through childhood as a genuine girl."

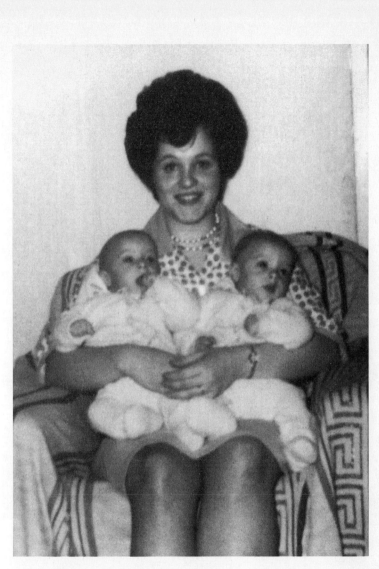

Janet with her twin baby boys, Brian and Bruce. The cataclysmic accident that would lead to Bruce's sex change was still some months in the future. *(Photo courtesy of the Reimer family)*

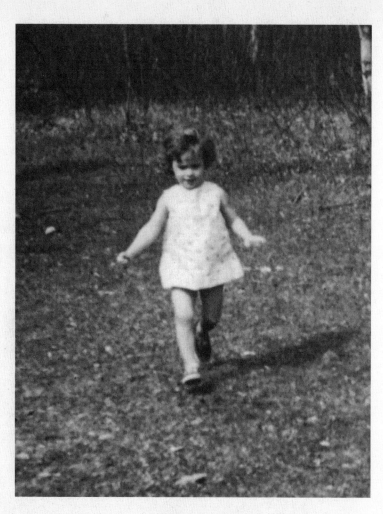

Brenda at age two, shortly after her surgical sex reassignment.
(Photo courtesy of the Reimer family)

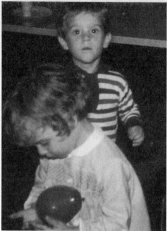

Brenda and Brian as toddlers.
(Photo courtesy of the Reimer family)

Brian and Brenda around the time that they started kindergarten. *(Photo courtesy of the Reimer family)*

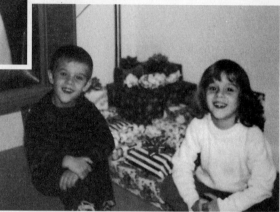

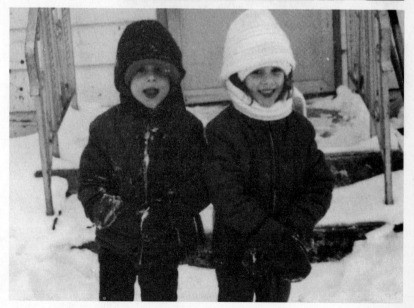

Brian and Brenda Reimer—the ultimate "matched pair."
(Photo courtesy of the Reimer family)

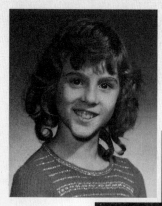

Brenda at age ten. "Everyone is telling you that you're a girl," David would later say, "but you say to yourself, 'I don't feel like a girl.'" *(Photo courtesy of the Reimer family)*

Christmas, mid-1970s, with Brenda dressed in her best clothes for visiting her paternal grandparents. *(Photo courtesy of the Reimer family)*

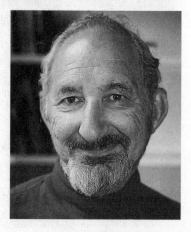

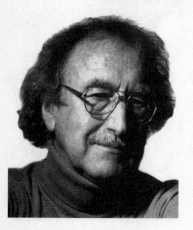

Dr. John Money
(Photo by Mike Mitchell)

Dr. Milton Diamond
(Photo by Sara Diamond)

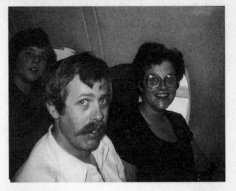

Brian, Ron, and Janet on their way to what would be the family's final trip to Baltimore, in May 1978. Brenda, the photographer, was careful to stay on the opposite side of the lens at this stage of her life. *(Photo courtesy of the Reimer family)*

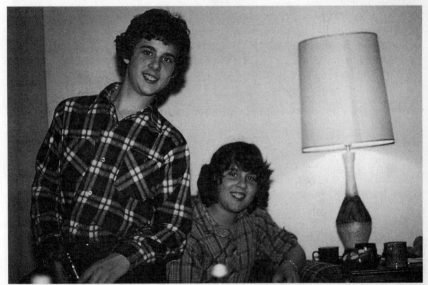

Brian and Brenda at age fourteen, shortly before they were told the truth of Brenda's birth. *(Photo courtesy of the Reimer family)*

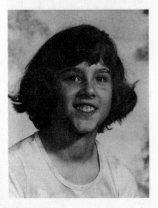

Brenda at age twelve, shortly after she started estrogen therapy to promote the feminization of her figure.
(Photo courtesy of the Reimer family)

David and Brian in May 1980 at their uncle's wedding, where David made his public debut as a boy. David still carries the evidence of the binge-eating he had done, as Brenda, to disguise his breasts. They would be surgically removed five months later, and testosterone injections would soon make David catch up in height to his twin. *(Photo courtesy of the Reimer family)*

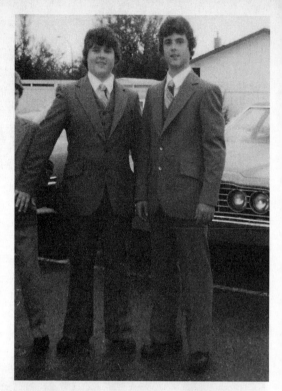

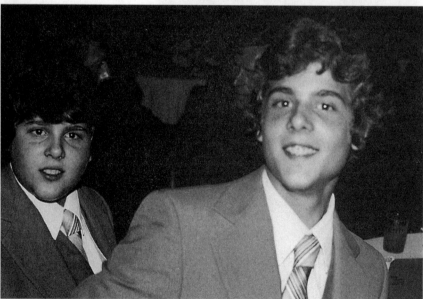

David and Brian, May 1980, at their uncle's wedding.
(Photo courtesy of the Reimer family)

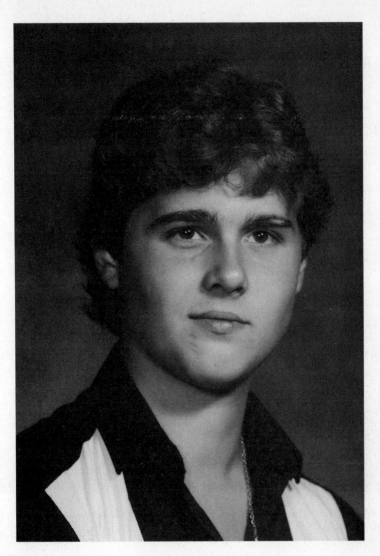

David at age eighteen.
(Photo courtesy of the Reimer family)

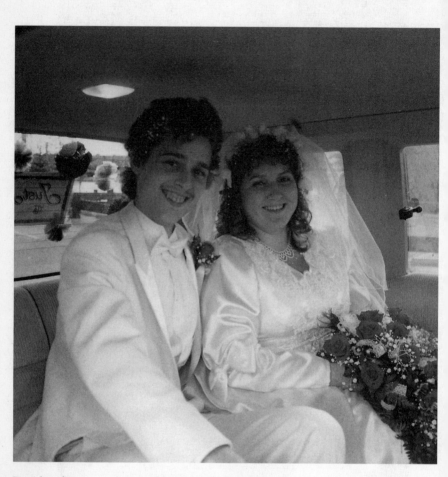

David and Jane on their wedding day, 22 September 1990. It was Jane's reaction to the truth about David's past that convinced him of her "true heart." *(Photo courtesy of the Reimer family)*

PART TWO

To Know My Birth

7

≡

THE REIMERS ARRIVED back in Winnipeg in mid-November 1976 and began trying to rebuild their lives. Janet found work as a cashier at a five-and-dime, and Ron took a job with a food company driving a lunch truck—a job he would soon leave to start his own business. Living temporarily out of the Capri Motel in the city's East End, the Reimers enrolled Brenda and Brian in Agassiz Drive Elementary, a small school located nearby on the edge of the comfortable middle-class neighborhood of College Heights. Up to this point Brenda's sole psychological therapy had been the counseling sessions during her annual visits to Johns Hopkins. This changed when she entered Agassiz Drive, where her anxiety, social isolation, and fear immediately drew the attention of the school's principal, Mr. Bergmann, who once again notified the city's Child Guidance Clinic. Joan Nebbs, the reading clinician who had handled Brenda's case a year and a half earlier, interviewed Brenda again in the fall of 1976.

"Brenda's interests are strongly masculine," Nebbs wrote in her new report on Brenda at age eleven. "She has marvelous plans for building tree houses, go-carts with CB radios, model gas airplanes. . . . [S]he appears to be more competitive and aggressive than her brother and is much more untidy both at home and at school." A session with the clinic's psychologist revealed that Brenda had "strong fears that something has been done to her genital organs" and that she had "some suicidal thoughts."

Brenda's case was referred to Dr. Keith Sigmundson, an amiable thirty-four-year-old who was then head of the clinic's Psychiatry Department. Born and raised in the small fishing town of Gimli, an hour's drive north of Winnipeg, Sigmundson had taken his medical and psychiatric degrees at the University of Manitoba in Winnipeg, then joined the Child Guidance Clinic, where his career ascent had been rapid. "Because I was just ahead of the baby boomers," Sigmundson says with typical self-deprecation, "I got a position that I was too young for and probably didn't deserve in the first place."

Even the most seasoned psychiatrist might have found Brenda Reimer's case a unique challenge. Sigmundson read Dr. Money's published accounts of the unequivocal female gender identity that Brenda had reportedly established, but from his very first meeting with the girl, Sigmundson was struck by her appearance. "She was sitting there in a skirt with her legs apart, one hand planted firmly on one knee," he recalls. "There was nothing feminine about her."

Sigmundson decided to establish a record of the girl's behavior in comparison with that of her twin brother and arranged for a clinical video to be made. Shot through a two-way mirror in a room at the Child Guidance Clinic, the videotape showed psychiatrist Dr. Doreen Moggey interviewing the twins. Or rather, *trying* to interview the twins. Brenda, whose yearly trips to the Psychohormonal Research Unit had made her acutely distrustful of any unfamiliar people or situations, immediately grew wary of the undertaking.

"It was a big room," David recalls, "nothing in it—just three chairs, one for me and one for my brother and one for this lady who was there talking. She had a notepad and she was writing. She was trying to get me to go over and sit down. But I was suspicious. I was checking all the nooks and crannies, checking the place out. I went up to the glass, and I saw the camera." Yelling at her brother that they were being filmed, Brenda immediately stalked out of the room and refused to come back.

Despite the abortive nature of the video, it did provide an accurate record of Brenda's mood, movements, and mannerisms, so that when Sigmundson convened a group of the city's senior psychiatrists, endocrinologists, and pediatricians to consult on the case, he showed them the video. "Everyone who saw Brenda that day identified that she looked like a boy," says Moggey, who attended the meeting. But in the conversation and debate that ensued among the assembled physicians, a consensus soon emerged that they had little choice but to continue the treatment Money had begun. It had simply gone too far to turn back. Nor was it lost upon Sigmundson that Brenda's case was famous in the medical literature. "I felt I had a responsibility," Sigmundson says. "This was *the* case. The idea was that we were going to try to make this work."

To promote Brenda's female identification, Sigmundson decided that she should be treated by a woman psychiatrist. He enlisted Dr. Moggey. A keen-eyed woman with a brisk, take-charge manner, Moggey was, like Sigmundson, troubled by the case from the outset. In an early meeting with Brenda, on 30 December 1976, Moggey noted the fitful girlishness that

Brenda (especially when under observation) could incorporate into her mannerisms and utterances—"a mixture of masculine and feminine gestures and characteristics," as Moggey put it in her notes. The psychiatrist soon grew skeptical about the degree to which Brenda's sporadic feminine adaptations indicated her sense of herself as a girl. In her notes, Moggey wrote, "One gets impression that [Brenda] sometimes says what she thinks you want to hear—'I am a girl.' "

As the sessions progressed, Moggey's doubts quickly deepened. She documented the way Brenda repeatedly voiced the conviction that she was "just a boy with long hair in girl's clothes," and that people looked at her and said she "looks like a boy, talks like a boy." At the same time Moggey noted that Brenda was vehemently opposed even to talking about undergoing feminizing surgery on her genitals and flat-out refused to return to Johns Hopkins where, Brenda complained, people looked at her and "a man show[ed] her pictures of nude bodies."

Moggey had read John Money's accounts of the case and was mystified. "When you read the papers and when you saw the kid, they didn't go together," she says. "That wasn't the child he was describing." Nor, Moggey says, did Ron and Janet seem to be the parents Money was describing. In *Sexual Signatures*, Money had portrayed Brenda's parents as blissfully content with the difficult decision they had been forced to make in authorizing the sex change of their baby. Yet in her own interviews with Ron and Janet, Moggey heard of the couple's recent near split, about Ron's drinking, and about Janet's depression and suicide attempt. Far from a husband and wife happily raising their daughter, Ron and Janet seemed to be a couple barely holding themselves together as they anxiously tried to comply with Dr. Money's directives on how to raise Brenda.

Just how slavishly Ron and Janet were following Dr.

Money's program was borne home to Moggey upon her first visit with Brenda at the Agassiz Drive school. It was a frigid December day, and all the girls were dressed in pants; Brenda was the only girl in a skirt. When Moggey asked Janet why she did not put Brenda in pants, Janet helplessly replied, "Because Dr. Money said to put her in dresses." Moggey had to remind Janet that Winnipeg experienced some of the harshest winters on the continent (unlike Baltimore) and that Brenda should be in pants like the other girls. Only then did Janet agree to dress Brenda more appropriately. Brenda began to wear jeans like the other girls in her class.

On 3 January 1977, a month and a half after she took on the case, Moggey wrote to John Money. She informed him of Brenda's behavioral difficulties and requested some background information "to help Brenda and her family make a more appropriate adjustment to her problems." She asked what surgery had already been done on Brenda (Money's published accounts had always left this vague), what operations were planned, and what efforts Money had made to help both Brenda and her parents "adjust to the sex change."

Money replied on 17 January and in a breezy tone professed himself very pleased that Dr. Moggey had become involved in Brenda's case. He explained that the second stage of Brenda's vaginal surgery had not yet been performed due to the child's "fanatical fear of hospitals"—a fear, Money wrote, "that I have encountered on only one other occasion in 25 years of work at Johns Hopkins." He added that mention of hormone treatments or surgery induced in Brenda a "panic so intense that it's impossible to broach any conversation on such matters without the child fleeing from the room, screaming." Nevertheless, Money continued, there was now "an urgency" that Brenda's fears be overcome, because the need for hormone therapy and surgery was rapidly increasing with her approaching adolescence. "It will be one of the best things you can do for her if you can help her break down this extraordinary veto," he wrote. Dismissing Moggey's suggestion that Ron and Janet had not adjusted to Brenda's sex change, Money added, "With regard to the help that you can give the parents, I think it is not so much with regard to helping them adjust to the sex reassignment, as it is to helping them adjust to one another"—specifically, Money added, by helping Janet control her depressive mood swings.

Moggey (having already found a psychiatrist for Janet, whose moods would soon stabilize with antidepressants) was nonplused by Money's reply. "I thought, There are more problems here than are controlled by the mother," she says. Yet inclined to defer to the famous psychologist's apparently greater knowledge and experience of the case, Moggey forged on in her sessions with Brenda, reassuring the child that she was indeed a girl and impressing upon her the necessity that she return to Johns Hopkins to undergo surgery on her genitals.

"But the resistance!" Moggey says. Sullen, angry, unresponsive, Brenda often simply refused to speak, scowling and directing her gaze to the floor. Mere mention of the word *penis* or *vagina* would induce in the child an explosive panic. Brenda remained immovable on the subject of vaginal surgery or returning to the Psychohormonal Research Unit. "Won't look at pictures of female bodies with Dr. Money," Moggey noted on 20 January. "Won't accept going to see Dr. Money."

Struck by the obvious depth of the child's aversion and concerned that Money had not yet grasped the severity of the problems that Brenda and her family had been laboring under, Moggey wrote to him again on 2 February. This time she wrote at greater length and was explicit about Brenda's problems: she explained that the child was two years behind her peers academically and had not progressed well in school "from day one"; that Brian was "embarrassed" by Brenda's "tomboy like behavior"; that Brenda was having trouble making friends and talked openly about being different from other girls; that she was "not interested in developing female shape," felt anything to do with her body was "dirty," was still refusing surgery, and had expressed embarrassment about her trips to Baltimore where "a man [was] showing her pictures of nude bodies"; and that furthermore "she is saying no to returning to see you and threatens to run away if this is necessary." Moggey ended the letter by saying that despite Brenda's resistance, she was continuing to work toward making the girl return to Baltimore, "as I do feel Brenda needs to start her hormone therapy and start developing female characteristics."

Money's reply, dated 9 February, was brief. Failing to allude even glancingly to the many issues raised by Moggey, he simply reiterated his great pleasure that the psychiatrist had become involved, his happiness in working "in closest collaboration" with her, and his "great relief" that Moggey was helping to prepare Brenda for her return to Johns Hopkins.

Money's relief was to be short-lived. After two more months of trying—in vain—to convince Brenda to return to Johns Hopkins, Moggey decided that no amount of therapy could remove the girl's fierce resistance. That spring Moggey spoke to Ron and Janet about the alternative of Brenda's undergoing the vaginal surgery not in Baltimore, but in Winnipeg—a plan that would not only save considerable time, energy, and money for the Reimers, but also remove for Brenda the deep anxiety associated with her visits to Johns Hopkins.

Still Ron and Janet expressed trepidation about deviating in any way from Money's program. They would agree to it only if Dr. Money himself approved the plan. On 18 April, Moggey wrote to him again and apprised him of the proposal to have Brenda's surgery performed in Winnipeg—"unless," she added, "there is some particular reason for returning to Johns Hopkins."

As it happened, Money considered there to be many reasons for the child to return to Johns Hopkins. He outlined these reasons in a two-page, single-spaced letter that seemed to carry, under its surface smoothness, a strong undertone of desperation at the prospect of losing control of, and contact with, his most famous research subject.

"It goes without saying the Reimers have freedom of choice with respect to location of professional services," Money began. "I shall go along with their decision, whatever it is. Nonetheless, I believe their wisest decision will be not to lose their Johns Hopkins contact, but to work out a joint program of cooperation between us and Brenda's local specialists." Citing the "unique" benefits of the "close collaboration between medical psychology, endocrinology and surgery" at Johns Hopkins, which, Money claimed, "eliminates the possibility of conflicting opinions among experts not accustomed to working together," he also extolled the vagina-building skills of Howard Jones, the surgeon who had castrated Brenda a decade earlier and who was scheduled to construct her artificial genitals. Yet apparently aware that even his own formidable powers of persuasion were not quite up to the task of explaining why it was more practicable for the child to travel two thousand miles for a complicated operation requiring lengthy follow-up care (rather than have the surgery in a hospital just minutes from home), Money concluded his letter with a plea that regardless of where the surgery was done, he not lose contact with Brenda. "I would like to continue seeing her," he wrote, "on approximately an annual basis in the future as in the past."

Only when the Reimers saw that Dr. Money would not stand in the way of Brenda's having the surgery in Winnipeg did they agree to the change in plan. But on the issue of Brenda's returning to Baltimore for her annual follow-ups, Ron and Janet found themselves once again persuaded by Money's eloquence. They decided that if Brenda's fears could be overcome by the local psychiatrists, they would continue to bring her to the Psychohormonal Research Unit for her yearly counseling sessions with Dr. Money. "We felt like we had nowhere else to turn," says Janet. "No one knew us, or Brenda, as well as Dr. Money did."

8

≡

IN THE SPRING of Brenda's sixth-grade year at Agassiz
Drive, her case was transferred to a new psychiatrist when
Dr. Moggey, for family reasons, had to leave Winnipeg and
go to live in Brandon, a small town some fifty miles north of
the city. Moggey referred Brenda to Dr. Janice Ingimundson,
a thirty-two-year-old alumna of the University of Manitoba
Medical School. Ingimundson was a coolly rational Freudian
whose considerable wit and warmth were carefully concealed
under a scrupulously correct analytic detachment. Not a
member of the city's Child Guidance Clinic, Ingimundson
had her own private practice, which she operated out of an
office in downtown Winnipeg. Her first session with Brenda
was on 6 May 1977. She recalls being taken aback at her first
glimpse of the patient.

"All the documentation claimed that this child had accepted
her gender identity as a female," Ingimundson says. "Yet my
one visual memory of this youngster is of kind of a"—she curls

her hands into fists and bends her elbows in a boxer's pose—
"*tough girl*. A rather boyish-looking girl. Rugged."

Little that Brenda said in her sessions contradicted
Ingimundson's first impression. Though at times Brenda said
what she thought the psychiatrist wanted to hear ("I want to be
pretty; I'm a girl, not a boy"), in the same breath she would
inevitably reveal contradictory feelings about herself. She
defended her preference for boy's clothing, telling Ingimundson, "I like dressing like this. It doesn't feel right to be in a
dress, like I shouldn't be in one." Asked about her feelings for
boys, Brenda said she "wants to beat up on [them]" and then
added a comment that offered almost an embarrassment of
riches for a devotee of Freudian symbolism. If a boy "laid a finger on her," Brenda told the psychiatrist, "she would take her
father's ax and cut it off." When Ingimundson tried to touch on
the topic of vaginal surgery, Brenda grew especially truculent.
"I have decided not to have that," she informed the psychiatrist, "and I don't want to talk about it."

Troubled by such statements, Ingimundson nevertheless
took Dr. Money's word that Brenda had formed a female gender identity. The psychiatrist felt she had little choice. "I
thought, The decision has been made," Ingimundson says. "If
you open up this can of worms now and say, 'Maybe this was
the wrong decision'—well, who is going to *do* that?" Accordingly, Ingimundson (like Moggey before her) resolved to work
hard to assure Brenda that she was a girl and urge her to submit as soon as possible to the vaginal surgery. Yet from their
first session on, Ingimundson was uncomfortable with every
aspect of the case—and in particular her sense that on some
subconscious level the child knew that she was a boy, yet knew
she must not speak of it.

"You'd talk to her," Ingimundson explains, "and conventionally masculine interests would come forward. Which is not

surprising; you see that in girls. But her embarrassment—not embarrassment, but her *difficulty*—in talking about those kinds of interests was acute. She didn't want to expose them. She used to say she had a 'secret.' She talked about wanting to be a 'detective.' She wanted to solve the mystery. That's the therapeutic puzzle: she wants to know, but she doesn't want to know. People in therapy want to know, but they *don't* want to know. They want to know only if it's good news."

And according to Ingimundson, it was clear that Brenda had come to believe that the truth was anything but good news. Ingimundson continues: "Brenda was basically saying, 'There's nothing wrong with me, why do these people want to cut into me?' And in retrospect, she was *right*. 'I'm a boy, I'm a male, so in that sense, there's nothing wrong with me; but anatomically, if I'm a girl, then there *is* something wrong with me.' So this is the bind that she's in. 'If I admit that I'm a boy, then I have to admit that there's something wrong with me anatomically. And if I admit that there's something wrong with me anatomically, *what happened*?' "

Thus convinced that Brenda's resistance stemmed from her inkling that she was not being told the whole truth about herself, Ingimundson, after their second session, talked to Brenda's parents. She urged Ron and Janet to begin preparing Brenda against the day when she would be informed about the circumstances of her birth, the accident she had suffered, and her subsequent sex change. "She has to be told," Ingimundson said, "and she has to be helped in accepting it." Only then, the psychiatrist believed, would Brenda recognize that there was no choice but to go forward with the vaginal surgery. In her notes, Ingimundson registered Ron's and Janet's terror at the prospect of telling Brenda the truth.

"I kind of wish that *you* could tell her," Janet said. But Ingimundson assured her that it was more appropriate for

Brenda to hear the truth from her parents. They should go slowly at first, laying the groundwork. Meanwhile Ingimundson would prepare Brenda emotionally for the final revelation.

A few days later, Ron had a private talk with Brenda. Sitting on the edge of her bed, he managed to choke out the statement that when Brenda was a baby, a doctor had "made a mistake down there" and that the surgery she was going to have was so that "other doctors" could fix up the "first doctor's mistake." Ron found it impossible to make any mention of Brenda's true birth status, her sex change, or in any way to explain what this "mistake" had been. Nor did Brenda evince any interest in these matters; in fact, her reaction seemed to suggest that she wanted to hear nothing more about them. As Ron later reported to Ingimundson, Brenda's sole response to his mysterious utterances about the "doctor who made a mistake" was to ask, "Did you beat him up?"

Today David explains that Ron's halting talk of an "accident" did nothing to tip Brenda off to the fact that she was a male who had been surgically changed into a girl. "You're not going to think of that in a million years," David says. "So I didn't know *what* he was talking about—and I didn't want to know."

Meanwhile Brenda was having her usual difficulties at school. "She has only been in the school for 4 days, and principal related peer problems," scribbled the school's social worker in Brenda's file. "Teasing—'looks like a boy, etc.'"

As the school year progressed, however, Brenda was gradually accepted into a small clique of misfit tomboys led by a girl named Heather Legarry, a short-haired brunet with an open smile. "I had been the subject of shunning several times throughout those early school years," says Heather today. "I knew what it was like, and I never would do that to another person—ever." Brenda, she says, seemed a natural candidate for inclusion in the group of tomboys who played soccer and dodge ball, climbed the jungle gym, and rode bikes. Though distrustful, at first, of Heather's overtures, Brenda finally dropped her guard and began to hang around with Heather and her friends. "Heather was the first friend I ever had," David says. "I didn't know what a friend *was*."

Heather, for her part, valued Brenda as a girl devoid of the duplicity and backstabbing that had poisoned so many of her relations with girls in the past and that even threatened the harmony of her current clique of tomboys. "Brenda didn't speak much," Heather says, "but when she did she was never vindictive or false. She was very honest. If she told me something was black or white, it was."

At the same time, Heather was not blind to what she calls Brenda's "oddity." Partly this was a feature of what Heather describes as Brenda's acute anxiety. "Brenda was always nervous about doing things that were the least bit unusual—like cutting through the university grounds on our bikes, which I did all the time. She was very nervous, very unsure of herself." Heather says that this nervousness even affected Brenda's speech. "Just making a sentence sometimes seemed hard for her."

And there was something still more odd about Brenda. "As far as I knew, Brenda was a girl—physically," Heather explains. "But from everything that she did and said, she indicated that she didn't want to be a girl. The other girls in our group were competitive against the boys; we wanted to prove we could do whatever they could do. We wanted to *show* them. We might get in arguments with the guys, but we wouldn't have gone as far as to fight with them physically. I wouldn't want a bruise on my face, for example. But Brenda fought with the boys. Brenda would take the bruises." Heather pauses and thinks about this for a moment. "I myself was a tomboy," she resumes, "but I never wanted to *be* a boy. Brenda did."

Heather's impression was only strengthened when, one day on the school playground, she noticed a small bald patch near the crown of Brenda's head. The hairless area was the result of an accident when Brenda was a baby—she'd pulled the cord of the electric frying pan while her father was cooking and been hit by hot grease. But that's not the story Brenda told to Heather. "She said she had deliberately taken a hot frying pan to her head to burn off the hair," Heather recalls, "because she 'wanted to be bald like a man.' "

It was through her friendship with Heather that Brenda became increasingly aware of a new and perilous undercurrent in the life of the classroom. She first noticed it when overhearing bits of conversation among the other girls—talk of "crushes" and "going steady" and "kissing." Then she saw boys and girls passing notes when the teacher's back was turned. Once she saw one. It was a love note, and it was signed "xoxoxox."

Brenda recognized in these developments a fertile field for fresh embarrassments and humiliations. She had resolved to give wide berth to the burgeoning dating scene—a resolution that she did not think would be difficult to keep, since none of the boys showed any romantic interest in her. Still, it soon became clear to her that she could not avoid the awakening sexuality of her peers entirely. That fall Heather took Brenda along to a birthday party for one of their classmates. The party began innocuously enough. With their host's parents acting as chaperones, the children dutifully played games of pin the tail on the donkey and Twister while a children's album played on the stereo. But when the parents left the room and went downstairs, everything changed.

"One of the kids took the record off—*zzzzt!*—and put on a makeout tune," David recalls. "Another guy put the lights out. Suddenly everyone's slow dancing and making out. I'm looking at Heather, and Heather was looking at me. We were the only two left over." The pair beat a quick retreat downstairs. "But you could hear through the vents," David says. "I could sense what was going on."

I asked David how he had felt as Brenda, watching his classmates pair off romantically. He thought for a moment. "I guess envious," he said finally. "These people looked like they knew where they belonged. There was no place for me to feel comfortable with anybody or anything."

Brenda's escalating alienation was clear in her sessions with Dr. Ingimundson, who continued doggedly to try to get Brenda to open up and discuss her genitals and to agree, finally, to surgery. But Brenda could not be budged.

"Not responsive to my efforts to engage," the psychiatrist wrote, when she and Brenda were three months into their sessions. "Silent . . . staring off into space—head turned away. . . . Telling me she feels trapped in office—wants to get out—or feels trapped inside self."

9

≡

IN THE SUMMER OF 1977, Brenda suddenly had to fend off an attack on a new front. On her last several trips to Baltimore, Dr. Money had spoken to her about the medication she would soon need in order to become a "normal girl." He was talking about estrogens, the female hormones that would simulate the effects of female puberty on Brenda's broad-shouldered, narrow-hipped boy's physique. Like the vaginal surgery, the prospect of growing breasts struck Brenda as a nightmare. So she was suspicious when one day soon after the end of her sixth-grade year at Agassiz Drive, her father produced a package of pills and told her to start taking them.

"What's this medicine for?" she asked.

Ron, struggling for the best way to put it, finally came up with, "It's to make you wear a bra."

"I said, 'I don't wanna wear a bra!' " David recalls. "I threw a fit."

The depths of Brenda's resistance to the hormones was clear in her dealings with the doctor whose specific job it was to prescribe and regulate her estrogen therapy—a pediatric endocrinologist named Jeremy Winter. A thirty-four-year-old professor at the Children's Hospital of Winnipeg, Winter had trained in Philadelphia under the respected endocrinologist Alfred Bongiovanni, who himself had trained at Johns Hopkins under Lawson Wilkins.

Given this academic pedigree, it was perhaps not surprising that Winter was the Winnipeg doctor least inclined to question the methods or conclusions of Money's twins case. Before meeting Brenda, he anticipated no problems with the treatment.

"I got the chart and looked at all the background information that was available," says Winter. "I read *Man & Woman, Boy & Girl*, and I believed it. I said, 'That makes sense, and everything fits, and I'm going to see this kid, and this is what we're going to do' "—namely, put the child on a course of estrogens and commence vaginal surgery immediately. But things did not work out that way.

"It was easily the most frustrating case we had in the clinic," Winter says. "We prided ourselves on excellent rapport with patients, being able to sit down with kids and talk and listen in a warm atmosphere. And here was this absolutely silent, angry child who didn't want to be there. I'd ask, 'Will you allow a blood test?' 'No.' 'Will you allow me to examine you?' 'No.' So I would have these monologues about the importance of taking the estrogen and having the vaginal surgery and how successful and wonderful this was going to be."

According to Winter, Brenda was especially adamant about never returning to Johns Hopkins. "I'd never seen a patient in my life who behaved that way about going to another doctor—who showed that depth of emotion," Winter recalls. Meanwhile, Winter had no choice but to try to get her to take the estrogen pills—an increasingly urgent need, since her twelfth birthday was approaching in late August.

Brenda continued trying to resist, but after continued entreaties from Winter, her parents, and Dr. Ingimundson (not to mention the threat that Dr. Money had once introduced into Brenda's head, that she would grow disproportionate limbs if she failed to take the drugs), she finally—on the eve of her twelfth birthday—began to take the pills. Or rather, she pretended to. When her parents were not looking, she would throw the small tablets into the toilet. "I remember the pink dye running out of them," David says. "I had to flush fast before my parents saw." Ron and Janet soon caught on, however, and took to standing over Brenda while she swallowed the daily medication—0.02 milligrams of ethinyl estradiol, later increased to 0.75 milligrams.

Soon enough, a pair of breasts sprouted on Brenda's chest along with a padding of fat around her waist and hips. The changes caused her deep mortification. In a bid to disguise the increasing feminization of her figure, she began prodigious bouts of eating. With several ice cream cones every day, her waistline swelled to forty inches. The added fat helped to camouflage her breasts and hips, but no amount of binge eating could hide certain other physiological changes that began to accelerate within her that fall. "Spontaneously expressed anxiety about her voice," Ingimundson wrote in her September session notes. "Starting to crack."

The dramatic deepening of Brenda's voice was a phenomenon endocrinologist Winter was at a loss to explain. Given her absence of testicles (the primary male hormone-secreting endocrine gland) and her estrogen therapy, her voice, by all known medical criteria, should not have undergone a virilizing change at puberty. Today Winter suggests that Brenda's vocal cords and larynx were perhaps thickening because of increased androgen secretion from her adrenal glands. Whatever the cause, one thing was not in doubt. Brenda's voice now began to change in a manner identical to her brother Brian's. She asked her mother why.

Thinking fast, Janet mentioned the deep-voiced actress Marlo Thomas from the TV situation comedy *That Girl*. "She has a raspy voice," Janet told her daughter. "It's normal for some girls to have voices like that."

Armed with this explanation, Brenda started seventh grade that fall at her new school: Glenwood Junior High, a large public school some five minutes' walk from her house. She was instantly exiled to the farthest periphery of Glenwood's social life, where she took her place among a haphazard collection of the school's misfits. One girl was an intersex. Another wore a complicated metal leg brace and built-up shoe to accommodate a right leg some three inches shorter than the left. Another, Esther Haselhauer, suffered from Poland's syndrome, a congenital birth anomaly that had stunted her growth, partially withered one hand, and completely retarded the growth of her right breast. Esther remembers that she sensed an immediate kinship with Brenda.

"She was hard to connect with," Esther says. "But there was something that I just responded to. It was . . . I don't know, a sadness. She reminded me of *me*." At the same time, Esther was aware that there was a big difference between the two of them, and indeed, between Brenda and any other girl she'd ever met. "Brenda wasn't a *girl* girl," Esther says. Furthermore, being with Brenda evoked a feeling in her that was curiously like that of being with a member of the *opposite* sex. "It was a feeling of security," Esther says. "When I was with Brenda, I felt so safe. Kids would beat me up because I was so small. But when I was with Brenda, if anyone tried picking on me, she let them have it."

David says that he was grateful for Esther's friendship, but that their differences made it impossible for them to get close. "She was always talking about guys," David says. Asked if Brenda ever expressed interest in romance with boys, Esther laughs. "Oh no!" she says. "That would be unthinkable; as unthinkable as me, at four feet tall, going out for the basketball team."

Six months after Brenda began seventh grade, Dr. Ingimundson received a letter from John Money requesting a progress report. Money's letter arrived at a particularly inopportune moment—just two days after a disastrous family session Ingimundson had held with the Reimers. Her notes on the 20 February 1978 session make it clear that Brenda's resistance to the surgery had abated not at all in the fourteen months since she had begun psychiatric treatment in Winnipeg. Refusing to utter a word, Brenda had pulled up the hood of her winter coat and folded her arms across her chest. Pressed to say something about the surgery, she finally burst into tears, while the adults looked on helplessly. "Parents & I at a loss for words," Ingimundson wrote in her session notes. The session ended soon after that.

With this fraught scene still fresh in her mind, Ingimundson wrote back to Money. She explained that despite their success in getting Brenda to take hormones, the local team had made no further progress in the case. "[N]o plans for surgery have been formalized," she wrote, "nor, for that matter, have they been discussed in a tentative fashion." She added that Brenda remained "resistant to medical attention" and was "still refusing examination of her genitals."

How Money greeted this letter is difficult to tell. His reply was written by his secretary—and it was brief. "Dr. Money has asked me to write you thanking you for your letter of March 8, 1978 giving a progress report on Brenda Reimer. We are very pleased to have it," the note read in its entirety.

A more expansive articulation of Money's opinion on the case soon appeared in a chapter of the book *Biological Determinants of Sexual Behavior*, an anthology of writings on gender identity published later that year in Britain. Once again the outlook was sunny. A full-page photograph of Brenda and Brian (taken at their last visit to the Psychohormonal Research Unit) showed them standing side by side against a white background. Brenda wears a short patterned dress with cap sleeves, her long, well-brushed hair falling to her shoulders; Brian is dressed in a boy's short-sleeved shirt and dark jeans, his close-cut hair exposing his ears. A pair of large black dots cover their faces, obscuring all but their identical jaws, chins, and eyebrows. Nothing in the accompanying text suggested that, beneath the black dots, either child was anything but smiling and happy. "Now prepubertal in age," Money wrote, "the girl has . . . a feminine gender identity and role, distinctly different from that of her brother."

An attentive reader might have noticed in this update certain evidence to suggest a less sanguine prognosis for the sex-changed twin. Elsewhere in the chapter, Money wrote of further research he had done into the role played by excessive testosterone exposure in genetic females in the womb. Money now revealed that there was reason to think that such exposure affected not only masculinization of play preference, toy preference, and career goals (as he and Ehrhardt had reported eleven years earlier), but other behavior as well. "The preliminary evidence indicates the possibility," Money wrote, "that there is a greater incidence of bisexuality and homosexuality [among such girls] than would be expected by chance."

That Money's famous sex-reassigned twin had spent her

entire prenatal life awash in a full complement of testosterone produced by the fetal testicles (a complement of testosterone some ten times the amount experienced by normal female fetuses) might have led some readers to conclude that the twin, at puberty, would in all likelihood manifest an erotic attraction to females; but on the all-important question of Brenda's sexual orientation, Money (perhaps forgetting what he had told Ron and Janet about her lesbianism) professed himself unable to venture even an educated guess as to what her partner preference might one day be. He wrote in his concluding remarks on Brenda's gender identity, "The final and conclusive evidence awaits the appearance of romantic interest and erotic imagery."

In the eleven years that had elapsed since Bruce Reimer's conversion to Brenda, none of her local doctors had ever met with John Money in person to discuss her case. But in the spring of 1978, Jeremy Winter was invited to deliver a lecture at the Johns Hopkins Medical School's Reproductive Biology Seminar. While in Baltimore, Winter arranged to speak with Money. Their meeting took place at the Psychohormonal Research Unit on 4 April. Winter detailed for Money the extreme difficulty the local treatment team was having in implementing his plans for Brenda: she continued to refuse to submit to a genital exam; refused even to discuss the issue of vaginal surgery; refused to return to Baltimore; and often refused to take her hormone pills. According to Winter, Dr. Money was wholly unconcerned by the issues he raised.

"He was supremely confident," Winter says. "Everything was perfect; there were no problems—and any concerns that I was raising were my naïveté and youth coming to the fore; and I would learn, in time, that everything was fine."

Money's own notes on the encounter confirm Winter's

impression. Money refers confidently to the time when Brenda will be able to "negotiate the decision [for surgery] herself"; alludes to his belief that Brenda's "intense phobia of white coats and doctors" reflects only a deep-seated sense memory of her circumcision accident at eight months of age; and opines, "I rather strongly suspect that Brenda already knows that she once had a penis and probably that she had been considered [sic] a boy." Still, this suspicion did not diminish Money's belief that Brenda would soon agree to vaginal surgery—possibly even at Johns Hopkins. As his notes show, Money also told Winter about Brenda's "intense rejection of any conversation regarding matters sexual, and of looking at books pertaining to any aspect of sex education." According to Winter, Money showed him some of the sex education materials. "He showed me photographs that he would use, dirty pictures, to see whether Brenda was homosexual or bisexual or heterosexual," Winter says.

Though unsettled by Money's seeming unconcern about the problems he had raised and troubled by the materials Money had shown him, Winter nevertheless resolved to feel encouraged by the visit. It was a relief that the world-renowned expert on gender identity did not consider Brenda's resistance to be an insurmountable obstacle to the eventual success of the sex reassignment. It was similarly a relief that Money, the world's leading authority on sex change, had endorsed the local team's approach to Brenda's case. "I was a very junior person going to the expert," Winter says, "and I was happy to get some reassurance."

But the dramatic depth of Brenda's resistance to Johns Hopkins and to the surgery was soon to be brought home to all concerned—especially John Money. On 2 May 1978, one month after Winter's trip to Baltimore, the Reimers returned with Brenda and Brian for a counseling session with Dr. Money. Brenda had fought hard against the visit, agreeing to go only when Ron and Janet promised an expensive side trip to New York City as a bribe. Yet even with Manhattan as a pill sweetener, the visit would prove so traumatic for Brenda that it marked the last time she would ever consent to go to Baltimore.

That something remarkable had occurred during Brenda's visit was obvious from a letter Money wrote to Winter several weeks after the encounter. Stating that "Brenda talked more extensively on this occasion than on her last visit," Money went on to say, "She was especially at ease with two youthful students doing an elective with me. She was quite explicit, however, about avoiding references to sex and sex-related topics, and to prospective surgery. . . . [S]he could not tolerate further continuance of such talk, and went into the next room to join her brother. I followed, and in bringing the session to a close, put my hand on her shoulder in what most youngsters would accept as a reassurance. She fled in panic. One of the students followed and helped her recover her composure. They walked, saying little, for about a mile." In concluding this oddly elliptical-sounding account of the events, Money referred to the student as "a woman." What he did not mention was that the woman had begun life as a man. She was a male-to-female transexual whom Money had enlisted to speak to Brenda about the positive aspects of surgical construction of a vagina.

The Reimers' trip to the unit had begun typically enough, which is to say, with Brenda displaying intense anxiety, anger, and depression—emotions that were reflected in the Sentence Completion Test she was made to fill out. "Compared to most families mine's . . ." "a loser," Brenda wrote. "I think most girls . . ." "aren't very nice." "I believe most women . . ." "aren't very nice either." "My feelings about married life are . . ." "rotten." "If I had sex relations . . ." "I wouldn't like it. Same if a boy would kiss me." "To me the future looks . . ." "bad."

But it was when Dr. Money introduced her to the transexual that Brenda's typically despairing mood turned to pure, deep-running panic.

"Dr. Money said, 'I've got someone for you to talk to who's been through what you're going to be going through,'" David recalls. Brenda was ushered into the presence of a person whom she immediately identified as a man wearing makeup, dressed in women's clothing, with a woman's hairstyle. When the person spoke, it was in a breathy, artificially high-pitched voice. "He's telling me about the surgery," David says, "how fantastic it was for him, and how his life turned out beautifully."

Brenda sat immobile, silent, apparently listening. But the words reached her through a clamoring, rising terror in her mind. "I was thinking, '*I'm* going to end up like that?'" David says.

When the transexual finished speaking, she led Brenda back into Dr. Money's office, where he sat waiting for her at his desk. Brenda sat in the armchair beside Money's desk. The transexual sat on the adjacent sofa. Money's transcripts of the meeting record what happened next.

"You do not have to have the operation for your sex organs if you don't want it," Money said. "And you can also change your mind and have it anytime you want to, whether you're in your twenties, or your thirties, or whatever. But from now on you're old enough to sign your own operative permit, and nobody can make you have an operation. As a matter of fact, nobody can make you take pills if you don't want. And you know that very well, because all you have to do is tell lies about them, hmmm?"

Dr. Money talked on in this vein for almost ten minutes, shifting back and forth from trying to sound friendly and supportive to sounding threatening and angry. He said that no one should make her feel as if she were having things forced upon her—even as he relentlessly tried to convince her to have the surgery. He spoke about her "gender identity," saying that she could not be a person unless she had one, and then he was talking about the operation again, about "sex organs for a female."

Brenda tried to interrupt, but Dr. Money said he wanted to tell her "a very nice story" about a patient who had been born with "a birth defect of the sex organs." Money began to talk about "clitorises" and "penises." Brenda again tried to interrupt him. "Let me finish," Money snapped. Recovering himself, he talked on about how this patient had always refused, like Brenda, to discuss his sexuality when he was growing up. Money said that he had learned from this patient not to force children to talk about things that disturbed them. Yet at the same time, Money continued to press her to speak. "I want you to know that I'm going to be the one person in the world that you can tell anything to, because I'm not going to yell at you," Money said. "And I'm not going to tell you you're crazy. I'm just going to listen and be helpful and find the answer to it. And you can tell me anything."

When Money finally fell silent, Brenda had only one question.

"Are you finished?" she said.

"We're finished."

Brenda got up and hurried toward Money's office door. Money and the transexual moved toward her. The transexual was saying something about taking Brenda up to the fifth floor where they could be alone. Dr. Money reached out for her. She felt the psychologist's fingers grasp her shoulder. Convinced that they were going to drag her off to the operating room, Brenda wrenched free of Money's grasp. Today

David cannot recall how he got out of Money's office. "I remember running," David says, "that's all."

"I heard the door slam open," says Brian, who was sitting in the waiting room, "and—*whoosh!*—there goes Brenda. Bolted. I hear John Money yelling. I see a bunch of people with lab coats running after her."

Janet and Ron, who were being interviewed in a nearby office, heard the commotion and came out into the corridor. "Dr. Money took off," Janet says. "We stayed with his assistants, waiting, while he went chasing."

Brenda ran blindly until she reached a set of stairs, which she dashed up, emerging onto a rooftop. The transexual had followed. Brenda crouched by a low brick wall that ran around the perimeter of the roof, trying to hide. David cannot recall what happened next. A report filed by the transexual (whose name has been whited out in the Psychohormonal Research Unit record) reveals that Brenda, with her pursuer close behind, fled down four flights of stairs and ran out of the hospital's back exit into a parking lot. The transexual searched the hospital grounds—then spotted Brenda running into the main entrance. She gave chase but once again lost sight of Brenda.

At the front desk, the transexual phoned Money at his office, gave a progress report on the search, then staked out the exit. Brenda appeared two minutes later heading for the door. The transexual intercepted her and offered to walk with her to calm her down. Brenda agreed only if they did not talk or come close to each other. "We walked," the transexual's notes continue, "Brenda about 4 feet behind me." It was in this strange configuration that Brenda and her would-be counselor proceeded silently some eight blocks from the hospital, then back again.

On their return to the hospital, they were met at the main

entrance by Viola Lewis—one of the few unit workers Brenda even remotely trusted. Lewis escorted the child to the nearby Sheraton Hotel, where Ron and Janet had been convinced to go and wait for her return.

Reunited finally with her parents and brother in their hotel room, Brenda told Janet that if ever again forced to see Dr. Money, she would kill herself.

10

≡

UPON THEIR RETURN to Winnipeg from Baltimore, the
Reimers found themselves enmeshed in a new crisis involving
their daughter—although this time the drama did not directly
include Brenda herself but rather the members of her local
treatment team. Several weeks earlier, Dr. Ingimundson had
terminated treatment with Brenda to take a leave of absence
from her practice and have a baby. Ingimundson had referred
Brenda to another psychiatrist, Dr. Sheila Cantor. An aggressive and outspoken woman, Cantor had taken a view of
Brenda's case quite out of synch with that held by the rest of
the local treatment team. After taking a look at Brenda's
medical records and Child Guidance Clinic reports and having one joint session with Brenda and her parents, Cantor
abruptly announced to the Reimers that Brenda's sex reassignment was a dismal failure and that the child must be
allowed to switch sex immediately to boyhood.

Sigmundson says that such bluntness was typical of Cantor (who has since died of cancer). "She was a good psychiatrist, but so strongly opinionated about anything she touched that she would alienate people," says Sigmundson. Cantor certainly alienated the Reimers, who still labored under Dr. Money's instructions to suppress all doubts about the treatment.

It was the ordinarily taciturn Ron who spoke up. "My husband got very angry," Janet recalls. "He said, 'First of all, we have to be sure that she wants to be a boy; don't just *assume* this.' He hadn't yet accepted that Brenda was not to be." Nor had Janet. Nor had Dr. Winter, who sided with the Reimers in their dispute with the psychiatrist. While Winter admits that, with hindsight, Cantor was correct in her assessment of Brenda's condition, he thinks the psychiatrist erred in her approach to the problem. "Even if you've got the right answer in medicine," he says, "part of this whole business is that you've got to wait for people to catch up and come along with you. And if you don't do that, the best plans don't work."

With Winter's support, Ron and Janet appealed to Sigmundson, demanding that he remove Cantor from the case. Sigmundson did so, which left him in a serious bind. Having now run through three of the city's senior female psychiatrists, and still determined to assign Brenda's case to a woman in order to increase her feminine identification, Sigmundson was running out of qualified women.

Even as the doctors struggled to find a way forward with the case, Brenda had settled on her own strategy for coping with her predicament. When Brenda started eighth grade at Glenwood Junior High that fall, Esther Haselhauer noted the stunning change that had come over her friend. Ordinarily Brenda was never seen in anything but jeans and a T-shirt, wearing no makeup. But something had clearly happened over the summer.

"I remember she came into the classroom," Esther says, "and she was wearing this matching checkered beige pantsuit with stripes, her hair was brushed, and she was wearing lipstick, rouge, and mascara, and she was carrying a purse. It was obvious that she was trying very hard to fit in as a girl."

Indeed she was. Following her last traumatic trip to the Psychohormonal Research Unit, Brenda had become convinced that the only way to avoid the surgery was to play along to the best of her ability; she would try to act the part of a girl; she would try to convince everyone that she was happy. That way, she reasoned, they might not force her to have the operation. And who knew? Perhaps they were all right: perhaps if she made a true effort at living as a girl, she would begin to feel like one. As David puts it, "I decided to play ball. I tried my guts out. I was miserable. I was unhappy. I was uncomfortable. I felt awkward as hell. But the pressure was on me. And I tried my hardest."

For Ron and Janet and the members of the local treatment team, Brenda's behavior that fall was initially a cause for considerable joy. "Parents have found her to be much more enthusiastic about school this year," social worker Downey noted in Brenda's Child Guidance Clinic file in early September, "and she has apparently been out shopping with some other girls." This expedition to a local department store had actually been at the suggestion of their teacher, Mrs. Bailey, who had taken some of the more sympathetic girls aside and asked them to help Brenda a little with her dress and grooming, which left something to be desired. Ordinarily her mother would have helped Brenda with her makeup and clothes, but Janet had recently taken a job as a parking lot attendant and was gone early in the mornings, leaving Brenda to fend for herself. Otherwise it is unlikely that Brenda would have been allowed to go to school in the ill-applied makeup and unfortunate beige pantsuit, which she had bought for herself while on a shopping expedition with Ron.

"The pantsuit wasn't exactly in style," Esther says, "and the rouge was in circles on her cheeks. She came off looking more like a clown."

David concurs. "I remember these girls took one look at how I was dressed, and they said, 'We gotta take you shopping!' "

On a trip to the Hudson's Bay department store, the girls combed the racks for Brenda and picked out a feminine-styled blue turtleneck sweater and a pair of designer jeans. After school, when her mother was back from work, Brenda asked Janet for some lessons on how to alter her angular, gunslinger's stride, which since kindergarten had been a source of such hilarity among her peers. Janet showed Brenda how to balance a book on her head to practice straightening her spine and smoothing her stride. "It was unnatural," David recalls. "I'd get all tensed up after a while. But you were expected to walk like that, so I tried to do it."

Glenwood Junior High held dances on Friday nights in the school gym. All the kids went; Brenda did, too. "I'd get dressed up in my unisex disco clothes—jeans and high-heeled boots—and tell my parents, 'I'm going out to forget about my worries and my troubles.' " But Brenda discovered that her worries and troubles did not dissipate at the school dances, where the gym walls reverberated to the taped strains of Rod Stewart's "Do Ya Think I'm Sexy?"

"I'd mostly dance with girls, in groups of four or five," David says. But Brenda also danced with the occasional boy. "I was *expected* to dance with the boys, so I'd dance with a boy," David says. "I'd ask some guy, 'You wanna dance?' They kinda look at you"—he wrinkles his nose—"and say 'No, no, it's

OK.' " On a few occasions, however, boys *did* agree to accompany Brenda to the dance floor. "Sometimes it was a fast dance," David says. "Sometimes a slow dance." Circling the dance floor in the arms of a boy, it was painfully apparent to Brenda that she was not having the right sensations. Instead of any romantic flickering, she felt only embarrassment and excruciating awkwardness. One Friday night, David recalls, a boy in ninth grade who was one of the school's main heartthrobs defended Brenda when she was being teased by a group of girls. Jokingly, the boy kissed her. "It was a peck on the cheek," David says. "I went home and thought about it. I thought, 'It doesn't seem right. I don't like this. This is how it's supposed to happen, but it doesn't feel *right*.' "

Such feelings of doubt, which Brenda had long expressed in her therapy sessions, had always been dismissed by her therapists. "These psychiatrists and psychologists kept saying that these were 'normal confused feelings,' " David says. "You have a sense that it's beyond that, but people are telling you what you're thinking. And only *you* know what you're thinking. It makes you feel even more crazy."

Still, Brenda persevered. That fall a group of girls invited her to a pajama party. "Someone sneaked in a mickey of booze," David says. "I didn't drink any. I faked it. I put it to my mouth, but I put my tongue on the hole so I didn't get any. Everyone was talking about *boys*—'Who do you have a crush on?'and all this. So I said, 'Oh yeah, OK, I got a crush on this person or that person.' I mean, what do gay people do when they're in hiding? They pretend they're straight. You toe the line, like everybody else. Act like everybody else, and you'll be treated like everybody else."

It was clear to Brenda that she did not feel like everybody else in the room. Especially when the other girls began to get ready for bed.

"A girl got undressed in front of me," he says. "I was so embarrassed I looked the other way. She said, 'That's OK, you don't have to be embarrassed, you're one of us.' She showed me her bra and asked, 'What do you think of this?' I said, 'I don't know. It looks beautiful; I like the lace.' And I'm sitting there turning red. I felt like Mrs. Doubtfire in that movie." Asked about any other involuntary physiological reactions that he might have experienced in the company of so many half-dressed girls, David smiles—and answers with an analogy. "If you lose your arm," he says, "and you're dying of thirst, that stump is still going to move toward that glass of water to try to get it. It's instinct. It's in you."

However, Brenda was now living a life in which every instinct had to be denied, repressed, hidden: at dances, at parties, in the classroom, and on the street. "I was like a robot," he says, describing the playacting that his day-to-day, moment-to-moment survival now entailed. "You're so careful to look *normal*, but you don't want to go overboard. You're saying to yourself, This looks like an appropriate time to smile. So you smile. This looks like an appropriate time to cross your legs. So you cross your legs. You're always thinking one step ahead, like in a chess game."

It was a chess game Brenda was losing. Despite those few girls who had obeyed their teacher's orders to be nice to Brenda, the majority of her peers continued to jeer and laugh at her. "It was sad, because it was like the harder she tried, the more she failed," says Esther Haselhauer. "The ridicule became worse."

Of Brenda's eighth-grade tormentors, Wendy Holderston, the popular and pretty daughter of a local singing star, remembers Brenda as an "odd duck," a "tomboy" who had "a deep voice and really deep-set eyes"—characteristics that resulted in Brenda's being dubbed "Cavewoman," a name that soon caught on among their classmates. At first Brenda tried to absorb her peers' ridicule in "ladylike" fashion, but one day she'd had enough. In the school hallway she rounded on Wendy, David recalls, grabbed her by the front of her shirt, smashed her against the lockers, and threw her onto the ground. Boys who teased her got similar treatment. "That's what always impressed me about Brenda," Esther says. "She'd actually fight with the boys who teased her. She'd haul off and punch them. I always wished I could do that."

David is more rueful when he recalls his habit as Brenda of beating up the boys who teased her. "It only made people think I was a bigger weirdo and ostracize me more."

By late November, the earlier note of optimism about Brenda's social and academic life had vanished from her Child Guidance Clinic file. "She has no friends in class," Downey wrote on November 27. More frighteningly, Brenda was also showing disturbing signs of deterioration in her intellectual functioning—a precipitous descent into a helpless, childlike regression. "She cannot spell the days of the week or the months of the year," Downey noted in Brenda's file. "As 5th grade spelling was too difficult for her, she had been placed back in a 4th grade program. She has not learned certain set routines in the classroom. . . . She has been waiting for other students to unlock her combination lock as she cannot remember her number."

David recalls the humiliation associated with his helplessness. "When you're going through what I was going through, schoolwork is kind of low on your list," he says. "The last thing on your mind is a *test*. You're thinking about survival." The Child Guidance Clinic's Joan Nebbs uses the same term when she describes Brenda's predicament: "It was survival," she says. "To get through the day. To get through the hour."

As eighth grade progressed, Brenda's continued ability to

get through the hour became increasingly imperiled. The more her sense of the disjunction between her physical and mental selves increased and her feelings of entrapment and confusion escalated, the more her thoughts turned to the ultimate escape: suicide. "I kept visualizing a rope thrown over a beam," says David.

It was at this critical stage of Brenda's adolescence that Keith Sigmundson finally succeeded in placing her in the care of a new psychiatrist, a particularly gifted and empathetic one named Dr. Mary McKenty.

Upon entering Dr. McKenty's office at the Child Guidance Clinic for her first session on 2 January 1979, Brenda was surprised by the sight of the smiling, elderly, gray-haired woman who welcomed her. She was dressed in a tweed skirt and matching jacket and stood no more than five feet one inch tall. "She looked like she'd be baking cookies for her grandchildren," David says. "She didn't look like a typical psychiatrist."

And indeed, Mary McKenty was not a typical representative of the profession. McKenty had always eschewed the strict Freudian rules governing psychiatrist-patient relations—rules that frowned on excessive personal contact, or even warmth, between doctor and patient. She had always preferred to use a nurturing approach that was, in part, a reaction to the circumstances of her own childhood. Born in 1916, McKenty had been reared in an affluent home (her Scottish immigrant father worked for Richardson's, the province's most profitable grain company) but one lacking in introspection and overt displays of warmth. "Her Scottish upbringing was not attuned to psychiatry," says Evelyn Loadman, who first met McKenty in 1934 when the two were among the first women pre-med students in Manitoba history. "But Mary happened to be the kind of person who was very sensitive to others and couldn't really figure life out until she started to think about what we are made of."

It was in the early 1940s, in her first job at the Children's Hospital of Winnipeg, that McKenty's unique gifts as a child psychiatrist emerged. McKenty made no apparent attempts to delve into the protected realms of her patient's unconscious. Instead she would come down to the child's level, playing games, encouraging her patient to draw, paint, and write. Thus lulled into a state of distracted absorption, children could reveal themselves by word and deed. Loadman recalls that McKenty's nonpressuring approach lent an almost magical quality to her ability to rid her patients of neurotic behaviors—bed-wetting, hair-pulling—that had resisted the efforts of other therapists. "She was the only one who ever *cured* anybody as a psychiatrist at the Children's Hospital," Loadman says with a touch of wonder in her voice.

McKenty was hired by the Winnipeg Child Guidance Clinic at its inception in the late 1960s and quickly established a reputation for success with even the most difficult children. Indeed, when Keith Sigmundson first inherited Brenda Reimer's fraught and complex case in late 1976, he initially tried to assign it to McKenty, but she was recovering from a double mastectomy and thinking about retirement, and she turned down the case. Sigmundson returned to her only in the fall of 1978, when he was unable to find any other female psychiatrist willing to take Brenda on. Recognizing that Sigmundson was desperate, McKenty finally gave in and took the case.

Ron and Janet formed an immediate liking for the calm, grandmotherly psychiatrist. Brenda was, by necessity, more circumspect.

On the one hand, Brenda was drawn to McKenty. She liked how the psychiatrist spoke in a kindly, conversational voice and refrained from scribbling on a pad. Brenda also liked that the bulk of her sessions with McKenty were taken up playing board games—Clue, Cootie, Basquetball, Sorry!—or drawing, painting, or playing tongue twisters. At times, Dr. McKenty would drop in an occasional question about how Brenda was feeling and sometimes *would* jot something on a pad, but somehow it was different when Dr. McKenty did it. "She'd be writing something down," David recalls, "and I'd say, 'Oh, you're writing something down again—spying on me, huh?' And she'd say, 'Oh no, dear, this is just so I can make sure that we covered all the bases, so that I can help you.'"

Yet on the other hand, Brenda could not afford to trust McKenty completely, since she had to remain alert to the nightmare possibility that the psychiatrist's friendliness might simply be a more diabolical tactic to trick her into the surgery. As McKenty's therapy notes reveal, Brenda used an array of strategies to see if Dr. McKenty's friendliness was genuine. She drew a cruel caricature of the psychiatrist and showed it to her; she seized one of the clinic's toy machine guns and took the doctor "hostage"; she wrote out a "Death Warrant for Mary McKenty." The psychiatrist offered no resistance. She carefully preserved Brenda's nasty caricature of her, even obligingly signing her name underneath it; taken hostage, she allowed herself to be marched at gunpoint around the office; and on Brenda's "Death Warrant," she dutifully filled in the areas where Brenda had left room for the condemned woman's vital statistics.

"I was testing her," David says. "She passed the test." Brenda dropped her provoking tactics and began actually looking forward to her psychiatric sessions with McKenty. "We didn't see each other as patient and doctor," David says. "It was a friendship."

Brenda was now in particular need of a friend, since an old nemesis was about to reappear in her life. That January,

Brenda confided to McKenty that she had snooped in her mother's mail and seen a letter from Dr. Money announcing that he was coming to Winnipeg. Invited to give a talk at the local medical school, he had made plans to visit Brenda and her family—a visit, McKenty wrote, that Brenda was dreading.

Over the next two months, McKenty recorded Brenda's escalating anxiety as Money's impending visit drew nearer. On 31 January, Brenda recounted to McKenty a nightmare that she'd had about Money, her twin brother, and herself. "Dr. Money was a magician with a cape," Brenda told McKenty, "and he said he could make us disappear—pouf!—like that. I woke up and thought we had disappeared." To allay Brenda's fears, McKenty said that she did not have to see the psychologist when he visited. Together they created the "Don't Want to See Dr. Money Club." McKenty signed her name on the membership list. Brenda added her own signature and the words "Join my Club!" But a month later, with Money's visit less than two weeks away, Brenda had another dream. "I had on a fancy blue dress and my good shoes, too," she told McKenty. "The skirt was split because it's too narrow. Everything was cleaned up—the floor was washed. Something big seemed to be going to happen. There was a closet nearby. We have a closet like that in our house. I was scared because it seemed I could maybe get put in that closet."

The week of 22 March 1979 proved to be one of those gray Winnipeg periods when the weather has stalled in the indefinable season between late winter and early spring. The snowbanks, having lingered too long, were blackened with car exhaust, and the sky was the color of cement. Ron, driving his Dodge Dart to pick up Dr. Money at the city's Health Sciences Center (where the psychologist had just given his speech), looked with chagrin at the dirty snowbanks. He'd been hoping for better weather so that Money might take home a more favorable impression of their city.

Back at the Reimers' house, Janet was having similar feelings of anxiety about the impression Money would carry away of his visit to Winnipeg and, specifically, the Reimers' home. They had moved into the house two years earlier and put two thousand dollars into fixing the place up. Ordinarily Janet felt quite proud of what she'd been able to achieve on her budget. Now she was seeing the place through the eyes of Dr. Money, whom she considered the most aesthetically refined person she had ever met. "The house had an old gold rug down when we moved in," Janet says. "It had been cleaned, but it just looked dirty. The walls hadn't been painted in a long time, and we had a cheap couch, an old beige sofa with an orange thread running through it."

By the time she heard the car pull up in the driveway, Janet had worked herself into a state of considerable apprehension. When Dr. Money stepped through the front door into the Reimers' modest living room, however, he seemed to take particular pains to project a manner of friendly and accepting approval of everything that met his eye. If memories lingered in Money's mind of the last time he had seen the Reimers—during the disastrous Baltimore trip the previous spring—he showed no signs of it. Certainly Ron and Janet made every effort to put the episode out of their own minds.

"He was like a friend—or an uncle—who had been away a long time and had come for a visit," Janet says. Dr. Money admired Ron's homemade wall cabinet and complimented Janet on her pen-and-ink drawings, which hung on the walls. Meanwhile the twins had disappeared into the basement and refused to come up and meet Dr. Money.

The adults sat at the dining room table, and Ron offered Dr.

Money a beer. Sipping one of Ron's Canadian lagers, Money relaxed and spoke about his childhood in rural New Zealand, where he said he had once seen a fireball and where the earth-quakes were so frequent that his mother had strung thread across her kitchen shelves to prevent bottles from falling during the tremors. Money talked about the dark beer that was popular in his native country and asked Ron if they had dark beer in Winnipeg.

Today, neither Ron nor Janet can remember precisely how it was that Dr. Money, who had planned merely to drop over for an hour or two, ended up spending the night. Janet recalls that Money glanced at the clock and announced that he had missed his flight; Ron thinks that perhaps a snowstorm canceled Money's flight back to Baltimore. In any case, once it was apparent that Dr. Money was stranded, Ron and Janet, out of politeness, invited him to stay with them—although they had only an air mattress in the front room for him to sleep on. To their surprise, the eminent psychologist accepted their offer. Ron phoned out for a bucket of chicken to accommodate their unexpected house guest. The children continued to hide in the basement. That is, until their parents forced them to come up.

During the stiff encounter in the living room, Money asked how the twins were doing in school. Brian did the talk-ing. He said something noncommittal about their academic accomplishments, then asked Dr. Money how he liked their city and how long he was staying. "Then," Brian says, "we wanted to go." Before the two could escape to the basement, Money pulled out his wallet. Saying that he would have spent the money on a hotel room anyway, he bestowed on the chil-dren fifteen dollars each. The twins then hurried back down-stairs. They did not emerge until the next morning, when Dr. Money had left for the airport. It was the last time the Reimers would see him in person.

It was not the last the city of Winnipeg would hear about John Money, however. After his departure, the *Winnipeg Free-Press* carried accounts, on two successive days, of Money's standing-room-only appearance at the university's Human Sexuality Conference. STUDENTS, MDs DEBATING WORTH OF SEX EXERCISE, ran the banner headline on the first day. MORAL VALUES OF LECTURERS QUESTIONED. Money had upset some students, the paper reported, by showing graphic slides of a range of unusual sexual behaviors. The slide show was in fact part of a standard lecture Money had devised to "desensitize" medical students to various sexual perversions, and had already generated fierce controversy in the local Baltimore newspapers when Money introduced the films to the Johns Hopkins Medical School curriculum in 1971. The show featured explicit photographs of people engaged in bestiality, urine-drinking, feces-eating, and various amputation fetishes. During the second day of his Winnipeg lecture (the paper reported), Money had also screened a stag film of five women and three men having group sex, then followed the screening with a speech in which he informed the assembled professors and first-year medical students that marriage was simply an economic compact in which the "heart follows the wallet"; that incest should not be prosecuted as a criminal offense; and that in cases where stepfathers sleep with their stepdaughters, the mother is often "happy" because she "is glad to have [her husband] off her back."

Dr. Robert Martin, a clinical psychologist and member of the University of Manitoba's Psychiatry Department, attended Money's talks. "He was a personification of the style of the time," Martin says. "He liked to shock, play the devil's advocate, and was very cocky and very self-assured. His attitude was very much one of bringing 'enlightenment' to the 'boonies.' He radiated that particular lack of anxiety that, personally, sets alarm bells off, and he gave the impression that he'd plunge into anything. He was not the sort of person that you would forget."

Steve Whysall, who also attended the lectures, agrees. A seasoned journalist who had worked in London's Fleet Street, Whysall was the *Free-Press* medical reporter who wrote the paper's accounts of Money's controversy-stirring visit. "I'd been around and thought I'd seen and heard quite a few things," he says. "But I was surprised that this [sexual material] came up in that form." Whysall was especially surprised by the deliberate casualness with which Money spoke about such outlandish sexual fetishes as feces-eating. He interviewed Money briefly after the lecture. "I asked him, 'Are you telling these doctors-to-be that they shouldn't be alarmed if they meet someone who comes to them with that kind of request or condition?'" Money, Whysall says, dismissed such queries. "He was pretending that *he* was shocked that I was so narrow-minded, so Puritanical."

Since the Reimers were not in the habit of reading the *Free-Press* (they preferred the tabloid *Tribune,* which did not cover the event), they failed to learn about the controversy their overnight guest had ignited. Brian alone happened to notice that Dr. Money's visit generated some media interest; while watching TV, he caught a snippet of Dr. Money on CKND Channel 9, but the glimpse was fleeting, and Brian failed to hear the gist of the report.

In the days directly following Dr. Money's visit to Winnipeg, Brenda began to make increasing strides in her therapy with Dr. McKenty—as if finally freed from the last vestiges of suspicion that Dr. McKenty was working in collusion with the psychologist from Baltimore. Arriving at her 4 April session from an Easter celebration with her family, and thus outfitted in full feminine attire—black cowl-necked top, garnet pendant, and mascara—Brenda pointedly rejected McKenty's compliments on her appearance, denying that she was even wearing makeup. At her next session, Brenda announced, "I hate dresses. I only wear them to funerals and weddings." On 4 May, McKenty wrote, "Showed me her purse and contents, which were a hairbrush, mascara, lip gloss and rouge given to her by her mother, but she remarked pleasantly, 'I hate that stuff.' "

It was the session of 8 June that marked Brenda's most dramatic psychotherapeutic breakthrough to date. That this was to be an unusual encounter is clear from the opening sentence of McKenty's notes. "Did not want to play any games," McKenty wrote. "Soon began to ask some questions about her medical condition." This marked the first time in Brenda's ten-year standoff with the medical profession that she ever voluntarily raised the issue of her genitals and the fact that they did not resemble those of other girls. Brenda told McKenty how her father had explained that a doctor "did something that was a mistake." McKenty asked Brenda what *she* thought had happened.

"I used to think," Brenda said, "that my mother had beaten me between the legs."

Keith Sigmundson was immediately informed, by McKenty, of Brenda's comment. The two psychiatrists discussed it, and they agreed that Brenda's statement about her mother seemed to fit with almost eerie neatness a central tenet of psychoanalysis: Freud's theory of the Oedipus complex—the developmental stage that supposedly marks every human being's psychosexual differentiation into boy or girl.

Named for the unlucky hero of Greek tragedy who unwittingly slept with his mother and murdered his father, the Oedipus complex was founded on Freud's conviction that all children, both male and female, develop in earliest infancy an erotic attachment to their mother—an attachment that eventually pits them against the father in competition for the mother's erotic favors. In boys, Freud postulated, the Oedipus complex gives rise to "castration anxiety": the terror that their father will neutralize the son's sexual threat by castrating him. In girls, Freud stated, the Oedipus complex breeds "penis envy"—a conviction that the castration *has already been performed*, that she once had a penis and has had it removed by one of her parents.

In normal female development, Freud argued, the girl's urgent desire to reclaim her missing penis compels her to reroute her infantile erotic desires for her mother and direct them toward her father so that she might, in sexual intercourse with him, take back the penis stolen from her, and it is by this means that she forms a "normal" heterosexual orientation. In Freud's view, psychotherapy was primarily concerned with curing the mental illnesses and neuroses that result in patients who, for a plethora of reasons, fail properly to resolve their Oedipal dramas in childhood. According to psychoanalytic theory, a crucial step in the resolution is to face the initial castration anxiety and voice it—as Brenda had apparently done when she described her childhood fear that her mother had damaged her sex organs.

On this basis, Sigmundson explains, he and McKenty hoped that Brenda's comment might be the articulation of a universal Oedipal fear shared by all females. "So we thought," Sigmundson says, "we were getting somewhere."

At the same time, Sigmundson admits that he was also forced to consider another interpretation of Brenda's comment—one that not only took into account the awkward fact of Brenda's intensely masculine behavior, but also acknowledged that Brenda *was* born a boy with a normal penis and testicles, which had (at least partly on her mother's authorization) been lost. Bearing these factors in mind, Brenda's comment could be seen to signal not an Oedipal breakthrough, but something less abstract—namely, the gruesome but emotionally logical explanation that a young child had used to explain the scarred state of her genitals and the bouts of depression suffered by her guilt-ridden mother. Viewed thus, Brenda's comment to McKenty could be interpreted not as her imminent acceptance of herself as a girl, but its opposite: her recognition that her earlier fears of maternal castration were incorrect and that now she wanted to know what had *really* happened to her; a sign, perhaps, that she was approaching the point at which she was ready to embrace the boy she had always instinctively known herself to be.

Whichever interpretation proved correct, Sigmundson and McKenty were now convinced that Brenda's therapy was reaching a critical stage.

The events of that June also brought Janet to a critical stage. Told of Brenda's statement, Janet was aghast. Already feeling nearly insupportable grief and guilt over her daughter, she found this latest piece of news almost unbearable. "I was just stunned," she says. "I couldn't believe that Brenda thought I could do such a horrible thing. I wondered, What must she think of me that I would do a thing like that to my own child?"

Today Janet cannot recall if this incident was instrumental in undermining her confidence in the entire experiment. One thing is certain, however. That June she and Ron were fast approaching the time when they would ordinarily start planning their annual visit to Johns Hopkins. Dr. Money had contacted them recently and pressed them to make an appointment for July. Yet when July arrived, Janet and Ron did not follow through on the plan to go to Baltimore. When

Brenda anxiously inquired of Janet whether there were any plans to return to Johns Hopkins that summer, Janet responded with a question of her own.

"Would it do any good?" she asked.

"No," Brenda said.

"Then we're not going." Janet did not bother to contact Dr. Money to cancel the appointment. The Reimers simply did not show up. Nor would they ever again.

11

≡

In the fall, when Brenda's psychotherapy resumed with Dr. McKenty (who, like many psychiatrists, always took a summer vacation), she told the psychiatrist that she had passed a boring summer at home watching TV and doing a paper route. Now, however, she was uncharacteristically excited about starting classes at a new school. The previous spring Dr. McKenty and the other members of the local treatment team had discussed with Ron and Janet the option of removing Brenda from the academic path and putting her into a vocational school where she could learn a trade. Ron and Janet, having come to recognize that Brenda would never be a scholar, approved this plan, and Brenda herself was enthusiastic about it. She told McKenty that she would like to become an auto mechanic—a job whose only drawback was that "no guy would hire a girl to fix his car."

In September 1979, Brenda, now fourteen, began ninth grade at R. B. Russell Vocational School, which was located across town in the scrappy industrial area of Winnipeg's West End. The brochures for the school had featured shots of a pleasant city campus; the reality proved somewhat different. A school that ministered to children with behavioral and family problems (some of the teenage girl students were reportedly already moonlighting as prostitutes), the campus, David says, was a forbidding concrete complex covered with graffiti.

The school had a rigorous hazing initiation week for freshmen. It was as part of this hazing process that Brenda was selected by her upper-year schoolmates as "Freshie Queen." On the day when she was to have the twenty-five-dollar prize bestowed on her, Brenda, as instructed, wore her best dress, a full-length gown with puffed sleeves and a ruffled lace neck. She then learned that she could not collect her cash prize until she danced with the "Freshie King." Her royal counterpart proved to be a small, stooped boy with a brush cut and a pained expression. The two got up and danced in front of the school. "It damn near killed me," David says.

The incident marked another turning point for Brenda. That September, after starting at R. B. Russell School, she took her sexual destiny into her own hands and simply stopped living as a female. Gone were the cowl-necked sweaters, garnet pendants, and purses she had adopted the previous year at Glenwood. She now wore a boy's denim jacket, torn at both elbows, dirty corduroy pants frayed at the cuffs, a pair of what McKenty described as "men's leather gloves," and heavy construction boots on her feet. She stopped washing her hair, which grew matted. Her voice had settled into the rumbling register in which David speaks today. Physically, her condition was such that "strangers turn to look at her," as McKenty wrote in her notes on Brenda. To the close observer, however, it was Brenda's mental state that would have drawn particular scrutiny and pity. For as photographs from this period reveal,

Brenda, for all her attempts to smile, had the eyes of a cornered animal.

"That was the worst time of her life," says Sigmundson. "R. B. Russell really brought things to a head in a way that may have taken much longer had she been in a more cultured society where the kids might have been more prepared to play the game. At the other schools they called her 'Cavewoman.' At R. B. Russell they looked at her and said, 'You're a fucking *gorilla.*' "

Despite the brutal intensification in her peers' taunts, Brenda refused to change. "I won't walk funny like girls do," she told McKenty—and she jumped up and did a caricature of a girl walking: "mincing along," McKenty noted, "with bent arm and 5th finger prominently displayed." Brenda enrolled in Appliance Repair—the first and only girl ever to take the course in the twelve years it was offered at R. B. Russell. The teacher, Hillel Taylor, was at first concerned about how a girl would fare with the boys in his class, but his fears were soon allayed. "Brenda could relate to the boys on a very equal basis," says Taylor, who has never been informed of Brenda's medical history. "I could picture someone like her making it in the military or something. I remember being questioned by my principal and other people involved—guidance counselors and so on— 'How is she fitting in?' 'How is she handling the boys?' " Taylor let them know that Brenda was adapting as if she were "just one of the guys."

Ron and Janet were not happy with Brenda's behavior, but that was fine with Brenda. "I was at that age where you rebel," David says. "I got so sick to death of doing what everyone wanted me to do. I got to that point in my life, I knew I was an oddball, I was willing to live my life as an oddball. If I wanted to wear my hair in a mess, that's how I wore it. I wore my clothes the way *I* wanted to."

And Brenda had more private ways of rebelling. Since earliest childhood she had been instructed both by her parents and by Dr. Money to urinate in the sitting position—despite her strong, overriding urge to face the toilet bowl standing up. Ever since she had been spotted by a kindergarten classmate peeing this way, Brenda had tried to refrain from standing up. No more. "If no one was around, I'd stand up," David says. "It was easier for me to do that. I figured, what difference did it make?" It made a difference to her peers at R. B. Russell. Caught one day urinating like a boy, Brenda was barred from the girls' bathroom. She tried sneaking into the boys' but was kicked out and threatened with a beating if she returned. With nowhere else to go, Brenda was reduced to sneaking out to a back alley near the school to urinate.

It was on one such trip that Brenda became conscious of a car idling in the gap between the houses that lined the alleyway. She noticed that the car had rental plates. The man at the wheel seemed to be looking at her. She zipped up her pants and moved away, but the car followed. Then she saw that the man behind the wheel was pointing a camera at her.

"I ran back to the school," David says. "I didn't know what he was up to. I *wondered* if maybe he was a reporter. You know that you're different. You go to the United States to see all these important people, so it's feasible a reporter would want to see you, but you don't know why—or why he's so anxious to get a photo of you."

The British Broadcasting Corporation's interest in John Money's famous twins case dated to some eight months prior to the day Brenda spotted the man trying to photograph her. Edward Goldwyn, an award-winning documentary filmmaker with the BBC series *Horizon,* had begun researching a film about gender identity in late 1978. A tenacious reporter with a background in science, Goldwyn had burrowed into all aspects of the subject, traveling around the globe to interview experts in the Dominican Republic, East Germany, Los Angeles, New York, and London. He inevitably heard much in his travels about Money's landmark case, which still stood as the single most compelling piece of evidence to prove the primacy of rearing over biology in the formation of gender identity. Yet when he discussed the experiment with experts, Goldwyn was surprised to hear rumblings that the case was not quite as it appeared in Money's writings.

"I was getting vibes from people in Baltimore being quite embarrassed by Money and the prominence of this case in the literature," Goldwyn says. "I could tell that these people were getting increasingly worried." They urged him not to put too much stock in the experiment until he had talked to the doctors in charge of the twin's care. Tipped off by a source whom he declines to name, Goldwyn learned that the child was being treated by Jeremy Winter.

Goldwyn contacted Winter in late 1978 and told him about the documentary he was making on gender identity.

"I was incredibly suspicious of some guy wanting to produce a show for TV entertainment," Winter says. "I was very frosty at the beginning." But Goldwyn quickly established his bona fides with Winter and showed him the extent of his reading and research. "He totally brought me around," says Winter. Having thus allayed Winter's fears, Goldwyn questioned him about the twins case. Winter cannot recall the precise words he used, but he says that he did disabuse the reporter of the notion that the case was a success. "At the very least, I'm sure I would have said, 'Look, I wouldn't take that case too seriously, because the reality of the child's psychological adjustment is really quite different.' "

Goldwyn wanted to know how different and was struck by Winter's reply: "He told me that the twin would have been suicidal if it hadn't been for Mary McKenty," Goldwyn says.

In January 1979, Goldwyn even visited the Reimers at home—a visit none of the family members can recall twenty years later, and with reason. Eager to see the family but concerned not to disrupt them by revealing that their identity had been learned by a journalist, Goldwyn settled on a ruse to gain access to their house. He declines to say precisely what his cover story was, but he says, "I came in as if I were asking if they could move their car because it was in my way. I was being, I suppose, a bit immoral, but I thought it was important for me to go and look and see for myself." Ron and Janet, he says, were "worried, lonely looking people." Brenda was surly, distinctly sexually ambiguous, and "somebody who I thought was really quite angry." In short, the family little conformed to Money's sunny portrait in *Sexual Signatures*. "Having found that the case wasn't a good data point—that Money's study actually didn't prove anything," Goldwyn says, "I felt the only thing to do was to leave it all out of my film. The only reason to put it in was to rubbish it."

This decision did not preclude Goldwyn's discussing what he had learned with a BBC colleague known for producing programs of a more controversial bent. Freelance TV journalist Peter Williams had recently been placed under contract by the BBC as executive producer on a new series called *Open Secret*, which was to deal specifically with medical scandals. Williams was fascinated by what Goldwyn told him about Money's famous case and asked freelance documentary filmmaker Martin Smith to direct a projected half-hour program on the case.

In late September 1979, Williams; his wife, Jo Taylor; Smith; and a small BBC-TV crew arrived in Winnipeg. Within days of their arrival, Dr. McKenty notified Sigmundson of Brenda's description of the strange incident in the alley near the school, where a man had tried to photograph her. Sigmundson immediately recognized that reporters had gotten wind of Brenda's location. As head of the clinic's psychiatry unit, Sigmundson had the most experience with the press, so it was agreed that he would handle the reporters.

"By that time," Sigmundson says, "there were *clear* doubts in my mind that this [sex reassignment] *ever* should have happened. At that point, I think I really wanted the world to know." Sigmundson agreed to speak to the reporters only under conditions that guaranteed the Reimers' anonymity. He demanded that the reporters agree in writing not to broadcast the photographs they had taken of Brenda; make no further effort to capture her on film; obscure the Reimers' location by omitting the names of all local treatment personnel; and finally, that the program not be sold in Canada or the United States. With these conditions agreed to by Williams and Smith, Sigmundson allowed himself to be interviewed at his home on 30 September.

Although appearing as an unnamed psychiatrist, Sigmundson nevertheless looked distinctly nervous as he faced the BBC cameras. Glancing frequently at a set of notes in his lap, he described the "significant psychological problems" from which Brenda had been suffering when she first came to his attention at the Child Guidance Clinic. He related the litany of Brenda's masculine appearance, her difficulties at school, and her failure to sustain friendships with peers. It was when Williams asked about the prognosis for the sex reassignment that Sigmundson paused. Several seconds passed before he spoke.

"When I took that long, long pause," Sigmundson says today, "I was wondering if I was really going to tell the truth or just fudge it. After all, it was still Hopkins. Money was the guru." When he finally answered, Sigmundson picked his words carefully, like a man tiptoeing through a minefield.

"I don't think all the evidence is in," he began. "And it may not be until she is a young adult that we're going to know everything about this particular case. At the present time, however, she does display certain features which would make me be very suspicious that she will ever make an adjustment as a woman."

Brenda's former psychiatrist, Doreen Moggey, also agreed to be interviewed. "I felt it needed to be done," Moggey says. "*Somebody* needed to say that this was not the rosy success story that was presented in the literature." On camera Moggey described the extreme difficulties she had faced with Brenda's case and recounted how she had notified Dr. Money of these difficulties by letter.

Ron and Janet Reimer learned of the BBC's presence in Winnipeg from Mary McKenty, who had declined to speak to the filmmakers.

"She called to say that there were reporters who wanted to see us," Janet recalls. McKenty told her that they should not feel they had to be interviewed, but Ron saw no reason to refuse—as long as they were not filmed or recorded. At that point Ron and Janet still remained convinced that Dr. Money's treatment would work, and they thought their testimony would be a help to other parents who might find themselves in a similar predicament. "We were too close to the situation," Janet says. "I had brainwashed myself. I couldn't *afford* to believe anything else."

In the Reimers' living room, Williams and his wife, Jo Taylor, asked how Brenda's treatment was working out. "I said I was still hopeful," Janet recalls. The reporters began to ask about Sigmundson's and Moggey's observations regarding Brenda's school performance and social life. The mood of the encounter changed. Janet started to cry, and Ron sank into a characteristic mute melancholy. The reporters asked to meet Brenda. Janet called her daughter in from outside and introduced the British visitors as editors of a poetry magazine that wished to publish one of Janet's poems.

Brenda, dressed in tattered jeans and a torn jacket, her unwashed hair falling in tangles around her face, stalked into the living room and said an awkward hello in her deep voice, then quickly disappeared. Her appearance seemed to make a strong impression on the reporters.

"When Brenda left the room," Janet says, "the woman got up and said, 'We're going to get to the bottom of this!' She seemed quite angry."

The BBC crew were headed for Baltimore. They had notified Money some weeks earlier that they were doing a documentary on the twins case. "Money initially showed considerable willingness and interest in being involved," says Smith, but that was before he learned of the reporters' investigative efforts in Winnipeg.

Williams and Smith arrived at Money's house in the early evening of 3 October 1979. At the time of his divorce more than twenty-five years earlier, Money had moved from the suburbs to an address just minutes by foot from Johns Hopkins, in a gritty, inner-city Baltimore neighborhood, where he continues to live to this day. "It was not the sort of place where you would expect a well-heeled academic or scientist to be living," says Smith. Money occupied the upper floors of a run-down corner store. Williams and Smith, admitted through a front door that boasted three locks, were no less surprised at the interior of Money's residence, which was decorated with the masks, totems, and sexual artifacts that also bedecked his office. Money himself was a convivial host—at least initially.

"There were a couple of his mature students around," Smith says. "We were having a drink quite casually in front of the fireplace and talking about the preparations for the interview, which was to take place the next day."

The reporters then eased toward revealing to Money the full scope of their documentary. "We think the case is very interesting," Smith remembers saying, "and we do want to do a documentary on it, but—"

"We should warn you," Williams recalls cutting in, "that we have heard other things about it."

Smith informed Money that they had spoken to the child's psychiatrists and that all was not what it appeared to be from Money's published writings. "At that point I think it's fair to say that he got extremely angry and annoyed," Smith says. "I think he felt that he'd been sandbagged into a corner. Which wasn't the case. In fact we quite deliberately told him that we had made contact with the psychiatrists *before* we did the filming."

Money, however, appeared to be in no state to appreciate such fine distinctions of journalistic etiquette. "His anger might have been that he felt that the child was being investigated or put at risk," Smith continues. "Or it might have been personal anger that someone should challenge his work. I don't know. But our relationships changed dramatically, and we were shortly out the door."

The telephone call to the Reimers' house in Winnipeg came later that evening. Janet and Ron had already gone to bed. Janet answered. It was Dr. Money calling from Baltimore, and he was in a panic. The content of the call has been preserved in notes taken the next day by Mary McKenty, to whom Janet recounted Money's conversation. Speaking of "persons unknown" but "suspected to be a Mr. Smith of the BBC" and another man— "a friend of Mr. Goldwyn"—Money told a wild tale of files possibly stolen from him and of reporters who had somehow learned of Brenda's whereabouts.

"He was all freaked out," Janet says. "He said, 'Don't

speak to any reporters.' " At which point Janet had no choice but to tell him the truth—that both she and Ron had already spoken to a man and woman from the BBC.

The extent of Money's displeasure was clear from a letter he wrote the next day to Sir Charles Curran, then director general of the BBC. After laying out his history with Williams and Smith, Money delivered a threat. "I would appreciate it," he informed Curran, "if you perused the contents of the program most carefully in light of the BBC's moral and legal obligation not to violate the privacy of a family which is at present particularly vulnerable to the possible effects of an invasion of privacy. I need hardly tell you that my concern is for the protection of this family. However, I must advise you that if their privacy is not appropriately protected I will counsel them to take legal steps to obtain compensation for any harm the BBC has caused them, and I trust that this will not be necessary."

But the BBC stood behind Williams and Smith, and the reporters moved on to the final stage of their reporting: to find a scientist who could comment on the significance of their findings. One name in particular kept coming up—that of the scientist who had inspired Money's wrath fourteen years earlier when he first questioned Money's conclusions and with whom Money had later clashed at the gender identity symposium in Dubrovnik.

"When we got onto Dr. Diamond," Smith says, "it was then quite interestingly obvious that we were getting into what is best described as scientific warfare—and that warfare can get quite bloody." Indeed, given Money and Diamond's long history as doctrinal adversaries, the BBC reporters were at first wary about using Diamond as an expert commentator on the case, fearing that any opinions he expressed might not reflect an objective scientific viewpoint. "You have to be careful to find out: Was this something personal, or was it not?" Williams says. "I was satisfied that Diamond was actually raising some-thing which deeply troubled him ethically. Whether or not he liked Money is quite another matter."

Diamond says that he had no special dislike for Money. Their altercation of six years earlier he had forgiven as a by no means rare eccentricity in a scientist and perhaps a result of the bibulous nature of the Dubrovnik cocktail party. Even after that encounter, Diamond had tried to communicate with Money. "I asked John several times in the late 1970s about the twin," Diamond says. "He didn't want to talk about it. He said that the kid was going through some troubles unrelated to the sex reassignment and that it would be inappropriate to bother her at this time. So I let it go."

But Diamond had never deviated from his conviction that sex reassignment of a developmentally normal infant was impossi-ble, and he had not hesitated to publish this opinion—even as recently as a few months before the BBC contacted him. In the 1979 volume *Frontiers of Sex Research*, Diamond had cited the case, saying that on the evidence Money had so far published, it seemed to be "good fuel" for the power of rearing over biol-ogy, but in what today looks like a statement of extraordinary prescience, Diamond warned, "with puberty, the penectomized twin has a good likelihood of rebelling at the assignment of rearing which is in conflict with biological heritage."

Diamond agreed to be interviewed, and his segment was filmed on a rocky precipice overlooking the ocean. Asked by Williams what impact it would have on the field if the twin were shown to be having "severe and sustained" problems, Diamond said, "I think it depends on who you ask. There are those who believe in the [case] almost as a religious entity." He went on to say that if all the combined medical, surgical, and social efforts could not succeed in making the child accept a female gender identity, "then maybe we really have to think that there is something important in the individual's biological makeup; that we don't come to this world neutral; that we come to this world with some degree of maleness and femaleness which will transcend whatever the society wants to put into it."

The documentary, entitled *The First Question* (in reference to the universal query at birth, "Is it a boy or a girl?"), aired in Britain on 19 March 1980. An impressively clear overview of the complex issues involved, the program also sought a balance in its depiction of Money's work. Included in the program was an interview with the mother of one of Money's intersexual research subjects, an XY male born with a tiny penis and undescended gonads, who on Money's recommendation had been surgically reassigned as a girl. At eight years of age, the child, Paula, was described as successfully living in her female assignment. Yet the program was unsparing in its depiction of the far more theoretically important case of the developmentally normal twin—whose case seemed to be on the brink of collapse.

Williams and Smith expected their program to stir controversy and comment. It did not. "The reaction was curiously muted," says Smith. "I was a bit surprised that print journalists didn't take it up." Diamond was similarly mystified at the failure of the documentary to provoke comment or follow-up from American programs like 60 *Minutes*.

Determined to disseminate the BBC's findings to North American physicians, Diamond wrote up the results of the documentary in a short scientific paper and submitted it to the American science journal *Archives of Sexual Behavior*. Titled "Sexual Identity, Monozygotic Twins Reared in Discordant Sex Roles and a BBC Follow-Up," the paper appeared in a 1982 issue of the journal. In it Diamond quoted Sigmundson's and Moggey's verbatim comments about Brenda's problems as well as Sigmundson's doubts that she would ever make the adjustment to being a woman. Speaking to the wider implications of the case and its apparently imminent failure, Diamond added, "As for the twin, it is scientifically regrettable that so much of a theoretical and philosophical superstructure has been built on the supposed results of a single, uncontrolled and unconfirmed case. It is further regrettable that we here in the United States had to depend for a clinical follow-up [on] a British investigative journalist team for a case originally and so prominently reported in the American literature."

Upon the article's publication, Diamond was frustrated to see it meet with a reaction similar to that of the documentary. While some feminist scholars quietly dropped the twins case from new editions of their women's studies textbooks, the academic, scientific, and medical communities were oddly silent about the findings. "They ignored it," Diamond says. "It's not what they wanted to hear."

In the days and weeks following her glimpse of the mysterious man with the camera in the alley near her school, Brenda grew increasingly outspoken in her rejection of girlhood during her sessions with McKenty. She complained of how Brian had more friends because he wasn't constantly being teased, and she railed about the fact that her brother could fight people without looking like a weirdo. "All girls do is make *babies*," she said.

At school, her "out" boyishness provoked escalating taunts and threats from her peers. One day shortly before Christmas, she was threatened by a classmate who brandished a knife. "I told my mother, 'I'm not going to that school anymore. I'll run away,' " David says. Janet supported Brenda's decision, as did McKenty, who arranged for a private tutor paid for by the government.

Away from the taunts and threats of her R. B. Russell class-mates, Brenda continued to assert her boyishness in word, dress, and deed while at home. Janet, hoping that Brenda's behavior was simply a "stage," continued to look for signs of femininity in her daughter. "Any little sign—and I was in seventh heaven," she says. "I misinterpreted a lot of things she did."

David remembers an incident from this period when Brenda found a pair of her mother's black kid gloves in a closet. "They felt nice and soft inside," David says. "I put them on. They reminded me of those cool Italian race car gloves that you see in the movies. I was thinking, These would give a good grip on the steering wheel. All of a sudden I realized my mother was behind me. I looked around and she was smiling at me, and she said, 'Go ahead. If you want to wear them, *go ahead*.' She thought I was trying to be feminine."

As the winter progressed, Janet found it increasingly diffi-cult to sustain such fantasies. One night she had a dream that years later she recognized as a sign of all she was struggling to repress about her daughter. In the dream Janet was visiting a woman whose boyfriend had just moved out. The woman, distraught, opened a trunk and reverently lifted out of it a huge stuffed penis. "She held it out to me like it was a brick of gold," Janet recalls. "And she said, 'That's what I've got to remember him by.'"

That winter, Janet began to feel returning the mood of deso-late hopelessness that had engulfed her during the family's ill-fated sojourn in British Columbia. In late January her psy-chiatrist, Dr. Nona Doupe, recognized that Janet was descend-ing into a serious depression and was once again a threat to herself. Dr. Doupe had Janet admitted to Victoria Hospital, where she remained for a month. Soon after her release, Janet spiraled back into despair—and life at the Reimer home fell into chaos. For Brenda, her mother's continued vigilance for signs of girlishness became intolerable; for Janet, the sight of Brenda in her boy's clothes and matted hair seemed an unspoken and unbearable rebuke for the decision she and Ron had made almost thirteen years earlier. In early March, McKenty noted Brenda's complaints "that nothing she does pleases her mother who criticizes and yells at her all the time." A few days later things reached a climax.

"She told me to clean up the fridge," David says. "I used as much elbow grease as possible, but it wasn't to her liking. I shouted, 'I'm doing the best I can!' She threw a box of cereal at my face. I threw it back at her. She was ready to hit me. I grabbed her hand and shoved her. My mother said, 'I'm going to tell your father!' "

Ron, pleading exhaustion, withdrew from the fray, turned on the television, and poured himself a drink. Janet recognized a return to the fatal pattern that had trapped the family in British Columbia. She called Dr. McKenty, whose notes on the conversation register the turmoil into which the family had plunged: Ron was drinking unsettling amounts of whiskey; Janet and Brenda were constantly at each other's throats; and now Brenda and Brian, too, were in open warfare, fighting all the time.

By now it was impossible for McKenty and the other members of the local treatment team to ignore the obvious: after almost four years of trying to implement Dr. Money's plan, Brenda and her family were only worse off. Dr. Winter was the only physician who still held out any hope. Convinced that the appearance of Brenda's uncompleted vagina was the chief stumbling block to her psychological acceptance of herself as a girl, he had long been the most vocal advocate for the surgery. But now, even he began to waver. "Early on, I had . . . pushed for early surgery," he wrote in a letter to Dr. McKenty. "I am not as convinced now that this is a good idea and therefore at the present time have no specific plans or opinions as to the proper time for the operation."

Ultimately Brenda forced the endocrinologist to come down off the fence. During an appointment at his office in mid-March, she refused to remove her hospital gown for a breast exam. The doctor asked again. She refused. The stand-off lasted twenty minutes. "It comes to a point in your life where you say, 'I've had enough,'" David says. "There's a limit for everybody. This was my limit."

Dr. Winter had reached *his* limit, too. "Do you want to be a girl or not?" he demanded.

It was the question Dr. Money had been asking her since the dawn of her consciousness, a question the local treatment team had badgered her with for years. It was a question she'd heard once too often.

She raised her head and bellowed into Winter's face, "*No!*"

To Brenda's surprise, Winter did not get angry. Instead he simply left his office for a moment, then returned. "OK," he told her. "You can get dressed and go home."

Only later would Brenda learn that Winter had, in stepping out into the hallway, spoken with Dr. McKenty. He told her that in his opinion it was time the teenager was told the truth about who she was and what had happened to her.

It was Ron's custom to pick Brenda up in the car after her weekly sessions with Dr. McKenty. The afternoon of 14 March 1980 was no exception. The only difference was that when Brenda climbed into the car, Ron said that instead of driving straight home, they would get an ice cream cone.

Immediately Brenda was suspicious. "Usually when there was some kind of disaster in the family, good old dad takes you out in the family car for a cone or something," David says. "So

I was thinking, Is mother dying? Are you guys getting a divorce? Is everything OK with Brian?"

"No, no," Ron said to Brenda's nervous questioning. "Everything's fine."

It was not until Brenda had bought her ice cream and Ron had pulled the car into the family's driveway that he found the words he needed.

"He just started explaining, step by step, everything that had happened to me," David says. "He told me that I was born a boy, and about the accident when they were trying to circumcise me, and how they saw all kinds of specialists, and they took the best advice they had at the time, which was to try to change me over. My dad got very upset." It was the first time Brenda ever saw her father cry. She remained dry-eyed, however, staring straight ahead through the windshield, the ice cream cone melting in her hand.

"She just sat there listening, real quiet," Ron says, almost two decades after this extraordinary encounter between father and child. "I guess she was so fascinated with this *unbelievable* tale that I was telling her."

Today David says that the revelations awoke many emotions within him—anger, disbelief, amazement. But one emotion overrode all the others. "I was *relieved*," he says. "Suddenly it all made sense why I felt the way I did. I wasn't some sort of weirdo. I wasn't *crazy*."

Brenda did have a question for her father. It concerned that brief charmed span of eight months directly after her birth, the only period of her life when she ever had been, or ever would be, fully intact.

"What," she asked, "was my name?"

12

≡

Brenda's decision to revert to the sex of her biological makeup was immediate. "When I'm eighteen I'll be what I want," she told McKenty in her first therapy session after learning the truth. "I'll go from girl to boy." The question was how to do it without creating gossip. She considered disappearing to Vancouver for a while and then returning as a male who had come to stay with the Reimer family. But there was an obvious drawback to this plan: "I look like Brian," she said to McKenty. "People will know." Then Brenda raised a still more agonizing problem. Trained her whole life to behave like a girl and to hide her impulses and feelings, Brenda wondered how her parents would take it when she revealed her true self. "What will they say," she asked McKenty, "if I go out with a girl?"

A month and a half later, the Reimers attended a large family gathering to celebrate Janet's youngest brother's engagement. Still living socially as a girl, Brenda had no choice but to go to the party in female attire: a dress, red shoes, panty hose, makeup, and a stylish, short, imitation white mink coat which Janet had bought specially for the occasion—and, perhaps, as a last inducement to Brenda to remain in the sex they had chosen for her. But the humiliation of parading herself publicly as a girl, now that she knew the truth, was too much for Brenda. Having vowed to change sex in three years, she now moved up the deadline. "In *two* years," she told McKenty a day after the party, "I want to look like a boy. I'd like a mustache."

At her next session, Brenda again moved up the deadline for becoming a boy. She wanted to do it *now*, and she told McKenty that she had been thinking about a boy's name for herself. She did not want to revert to her birth name, Bruce, which she considered a name for "geeks and nerds." She'd come up with two options. She liked Joe because it had no pretensions; it was a name for Everyman. She also thought of calling herself David, after the biblical king and giant-slayer. "It reminded me of the guy with the odds stacked against him," David says, "the guy who was facing up to a giant eight feet tall. It reminded me of courage."

Brenda left the final decision up to her parents, who chose the name David. Ron says it was easy to make the transition from calling their child Brenda and he cannot recall ever accidentally calling his son Brenda after that. Others, too, found Brenda's transformation to David easier to accept than they had anticipated. David's tutor, Dorothy Troop, says that she had initially been nervous when notified of the change, but when David arrived for his first tutoring session, Troop found that his maleness was far from an obstacle between them. Brenda had always been a sullen, depressed, angry child; as David, everything was different. "He was happier," Troop says, "far more settled and *alive* to what was going on around him." Troop gave David a chain with his new name on it. In return, David gave his tutor a gift: the imitation mink jacket he had worn to the family party. "He seemed to want to get rid of anything that reminded him of when he was Brenda," Troop recalls.

That August, one week after his fifteenth birthday, David made his big public debut as a boy among his extended family. The occasion was the wedding ceremony and reception of his uncle Dale. Using tape to flatten the breasts that still protruded from his chest, David donned a starched white dress shirt, a dark tie, and a charcoal gray suit identical to his brother Brian's. It was not easy, David says, to step out as a boy for the first time in front of aunts, uncles, grandparents, and friends. He knew that the whole family had been informed long ago about his sex reassignment as a baby, but this knowledge did not make it any easier for him, trained for so long to play the little lady in front of relatives. Still, determined to get up in front of the crowd, he danced with the bride and several of her bridesmaids. "Happy," Dr. McKenty wrote in her session notes with David two days later, "wedding a success."

David began to receive injections of testosterone. He soon boasted a growth of peach fuzz on his cheeks and chin, and he grew over an inch in height. On 22 October 1980 he underwent a double mastectomy, an intensely painful procedure that left him in agony for weeks afterward. He decided to wait until the following summer—until he finished tenth grade—before having any further surgery.

In the intervening months, he fell to brooding on the accident that had set his life on its bewildering course. "At that stage in his life," Dr. Winter says, "all he wanted was a gun to kill the doctor who had done that to him." As the dismal Winnipeg winter progressed, David's fantasies of revenge began to take on the contours of reality. With two hundred dollars saved from his paper route money, David bought an unlicensed 1950 Russian Luger on the streets of downtown Winnipeg. One February day he went to the Winnipeg clinic where Dr. Jean-Marie Huot had an office.

"I had the gun in my pocket," David says. "I opened the door to his office. He looked at me and says, 'Yes, what can I do for you?' I said, 'Do you remember me?' He said, 'No. Should I remember you?' I said, 'Take a good look.' Then he knew who I was. He nodded his head. I was intending to pull out the gun and blow his brains out, but he started crying. I felt sorry for him. He had his head down. I said, 'Do you know the hell you put me through?' He didn't say anything, just sat there, crying. I walked out. I could hear him behind me saying, 'Wait! Wait!' But I left. I sat by the river, crying."

David smashed the gun with a rock and threw it into the Red River. A few days later he admitted to McKenty that he had gone to Huot's office and "blasted him about the accident." He did not say he had been carrying a gun in his pocket.

I contacted Dr. Huot in the summer of 1997. He refused to speak about this encounter. "That was seventeen years ago," he said, "a very long time ago." Nor did he care to discuss the incident that had brought the murderously depressed fifteen-year-old boy to his office in the first place. Asked about the circumcision accident, Huot said in his heavy French-Canadian accent, "I'm not in a situation to start talking about that now, for sure, for sure, for *sure*."

On 2 July 1981, a month before his sixteenth birthday, David underwent surgery to create a rudimentary penis. Constructed of muscles and skin from the inside of his thighs, the penis was attached to the small stump of remaining penile corpora under the skin. False testicles, made of light-colored plastic, were inserted into his reconstructed scrotum. The sensation of a penis hanging between his legs was odd and unfamiliar. And he soon learned the drawbacks to phalloplasties. Over that first year, he was hospitalized eighteen times for blockages and infections in his artificial urethra. He would continue to be hospitalized regularly over the next three years.

Meanwhile, David tried to come to terms with his new life, and to prepare for reentering the world. In some respects, he says, this proved less difficult than he had feared. For apart from her fleeting friendships with Heather Legarry and Esther Haselhauer, Brenda had suffered severe social rejection; this, along with her almost annual changes of school, had guaranteed that no one ever got close enough to her to remark on her sudden vanishing—and David's sudden materialization. Still, after his reversion to his biological sex, David (fearing that he might run into someone who would recognize him as the former Brenda) took the precaution of lying low in his parents' basement. He watched TV, listened to records, and mulled all that had happened to him, trying to absorb and process it. This period would ultimately extend to nearly two years, until gradually, around the time of his eighteenth birthday, he began to emerge from the house, hanging out at local fast-food joints, roller rinks, and bars with Brian and his friends. Brian's buddies immediately accepted David as one of the guys, but there were inevitably kids who vaguely recalled that Brian had once had a sister named Brenda.

Together the twins dreamed up a story to explain Brenda's disappearance. They claimed she had gone to live with her boyfriend in British Columbia and had died in a plane crash. David was Brian's long-lost cousin. As for David's frequent hospitalizations, the twins said that they were to treat injuries sustained in a motorcycle accident.

"We all knew they weren't telling us the entire truth," says

Lyle Denike, one of Brian and David's friends from that era. "But we didn't want to push things too far. We knew we were dealing with something very personal."

Heather Legarry, Brenda's friend from sixth grade, also had doubts. In July 1983 she was working for the summer at her brother's Go-Cart track after completing her freshman year of college. "I was selling tickets," Heather says. "Suddenly there was a familiar face at the counter. It was Brian Reimer—or so I thought. I said hi, but instead of smiling, he flushed and stammered, then stepped away and pointed at this other guy. Up steps the *real* Brian. I asked, 'Who was that? He looks just like you.' Brian said, 'That's my cousin David.' I wondered if it was Brenda, but I just brushed it off, telling myself, If he says it's his cousin, it's his cousin."

"I couldn't say anything to her," David says of this encounter with the one person from his childhood whom he had considered a true friend. "It would take too long to explain everything. It was easier just to avoid people."

Later that summer, when David turned eighteen, he reached another milestone, for it was then that he came into possession of the money that had been held in trust for him since he was two and a half years old—money awarded to him when St. Boniface Hospital settled out of court with Ron and Janet for a sum of sixty-six thousand dollars in 1967. This was far less than the millions that some had predicted they would receive in compensation for their son's penile ablation. But then urgently in need of funds, and warned by their lawyer that a judge might overturn a large jury award, the young couple had accepted the hospital's offer. In 1960s dollars, it had seemed a considerable sum to Ron, who at the time had an annual income of only six thousand dollars. Placed in trust for David, the settlement money was to be used by Ron and Janet only for treatment associated with David's injury and had financed the family's annual trips to Johns Hopkins. By 1983 the money had grown to over a hundred and seventy thousand dollars—a sum that instantly made David one of the best-heeled young men in his peer group. In the hopes of "lassoing some ladies" (as he would later tell Diamond), he bought a souped-up van. Equipped with a wet bar, TV, and wall-to-wall carpeting, it was quickly dubbed "The Shaggin' Wagon."

David did not do any shagging in the van, however. Indeed it was in his relations to girls that he felt the worst complications of his transition—complications that were only exacerbated by the fact that by age eighteen he was not merely a passably attractive young man, but an arrestingly handsome one. His sudden popularity with what was now the opposite sex introduced a terrible dilemma, because he knew his penis neither resembled nor performed like the real thing (it was incapable of becoming erect). "How do you even *start* dating?" David says, recalling this period of his life. "You *can't*. You're in such an embarrassing situation."

Eventually he did date a girl two years his junior, a pretty but flighty sixteen-year-old. For David there was an ever-present anxiety. "I would think, What the hell is going to happen when she wants to go further than a kiss? How am I going to handle *that*?" He developed a strategy for stopping their sexual encounters before they became too intimate: he would drink a lot and then say, *I'm tired, I'm going to pass out now.* But one evening he miscalculated and truly did drop unconscious after drinking too much. When he woke in the morning, his girlfriend was beside him in the bed, and he could tell from her expression that she had looked between his legs. He had no choice now but to tell her. He explained that he had suffered an "accident." Within days, he says, everyone knew. Just as in his childhood, he was suddenly the object of muttered comments, giggling, and ridicule. For

David, this proved unbearable. The next day, he swallowed a bottle of his mother's antidepressants and lay down on his parents' sofa to die.

Ron and Janet discovered him unconscious. "Me and Janet looked at each other," Ron recalls, "and we were wondering if we *should* wake him up."

Janet remembers saying to Ron, "I wonder if we should just leave him, because that kid has done nothing but suffer all his life. He really wants to die." Within seconds, however, she had made up her mind, and they lifted him and rushed him to the hospital, where his stomach was pumped. On his release one week later, he tried it again, ingesting another bottle of his mother's antidepressants, then running a bath with the intention of drowning himself. "I was thinking, *When you're dead you don't feel anything, no pain in your heart, no pain in your body, no humiliation—nothing,* but I couldn't make it to the bathtub. Every step was like I had a hundred-pound weight on each foot." With the overdose beginning to suck him under, he lay down on the sofa and dropped unconscious. This time Brian saved him.

David withdrew from the world. He spent sojourns of up to six months at a time alone in a cabin in the woods near Lake Winnipeg. By now he refused to see even Dr. McKenty, but she had convinced him to bring a tape recorder with him to the cabin and to speak his thoughts into it. One night in January 1985, he did so.

"This is David Reimer," he began, his voice slurred with alcohol. "I'm nineteen. Soon I'll be turning twenty. I'm halfway through grade twelve. What I plan to do in my life is"—after a pause, he continued in a new tone—"OK, by the time I'm twenty-five, I should be all fixed up. I don't plan to marry until I'm in my thirties, because I'm just not the—not the type to get married." He rambled for a few minutes before returning to the subject that was preying obsessively on his mind. "I want to marry a chick that's sort of shy," he said. "Not *too* shy. And I would prefer her to have kids of her own. Because I want to have kids. And I can't have kids." This statement seemed to trigger a new set of associations. "Oh yeah," he said, "I got some money, about a hundred grand, because of an accident I had a long time ago. When I was small." He paused again, as if trying to decide whether he had the energy, or inclination, to speak about this part of his life. He did not. "Well, that's just about it," he said. "I hope everybody out there has a great life." He turned off the recorder and never made another tape.

It was not until almost a year after David had retreated to his cabin, that two friends of his, Harold Normand and Ron Mandel, talked him into leaving the woods and indeed getting far from frigid mid-winter Manitoba. Given subsequent events, there was an irony in the destination the three young men chose: Hawaii. On 11 January 1986 they flew to Honolulu, where they stayed for a week in the Outrigger Hotel not ten minutes drive from Milton Diamond's house. The trip had a salubrious effect on David, but it was an incident in the airplane on the way *to* Hawaii that suggested he was finally coming out of his depression and beginning to come to terms with the secrets of his past.

In the plane over the Pacific Ocean, he turned to Harold. "He said to me, 'I always wanted to tell you about that sister of Brian's,' " Harold recalls. "I said, 'You don't have to. I already know.' "

Harold had heard the truth three years earlier when he first met David. Immediately suspicious about the tale of the twin sister who had died in a plane crash, Harold mentioned the mystery to his parents. They instantly recalled the short newspaper item from 1967 about a twin boy who had lost his penis while being circumcised at St. Boniface Hospital. They had later learned through the grapevine that the family was named Reimer and had even heard whispers that the boy had been raised as a girl. "My parents put two and two together," Harold recalls. A uniquely private person himself, Harold had never gossiped about David's secret among their friends and had never revealed to David that he knew the truth.

In the months after their trip to Hawaii, David confided much to his friend that he had never told anyone except Mary McKenty. "He said to me that he never felt like a girl, so that when he found out he was a boy, his mind was made up to switch back," says Harold. "Either that, or he was going to be a lesbian. Because that was his biggest problem when he was growing up. He had feelings about girls."

After his return from Hawaii, David heard from his doctor about a new type of artificial penis, one that would, the doctor said, be a vast improvement over his current one. His new penis would resemble the real thing, and through the use of advanced microsurgery could be supplied with sensation. Shortly before his twenty-second birthday, David underwent a second phalloplasty. In a twelve-stage operation, which took three surgeons thirteen hours to perform, David underwent a procedure known as microvascular right radial artery forearm flap reconstruction of the penis—an operation in which the flesh, nerves, and an artery from his right wrist to elbow were cut away and formed into a tube to build the new urethra and main body of his penis, and a segment of cartilage was grafted from one of his left ribs to give structural support to the organ. Despite the long recovery time, David was delighted with the results, which were immeasurably better than his former phalloplasty. "I was driving down the street afterward," David says, "and I just started crying."

Despite the marked improvement in both appearance and sensation of his new penis, it would be two more years before David used it for sex. The delay had less to do with his feelings of confidence about his penis, he says, than with the legacy of what had been done to him in the operating room at Johns Hopkins Hospital when he was twenty-two months old—his castration. "I kept thinking, What am I going to say to the woman I meet who I want to marry?" David remembers. "What am I going to say to her when she says she wants children and I can't give her children?" Even if he did meet a woman who said she did not want to have children, she might change her mind later in life and then resent him. "I thought it would be *unfair* for me to do that to somebody I love," David says.

Still, David could not put thoughts of marriage and children out of his mind. His brother had married at the age of nineteen, and by the summer of 1988, Brian was twice a father—and possessed everything David wanted for himself. "I got so terribly lonely," David says. "I did something I'd never done before. I wound up praying to God. I said, 'You know, I've had such a terrible life. I'm not going to complain to You, because You must have some idea of why You're putting me through this. But I could be a good husband if I was given the chance; I think I could be a good father, if I was given a chance.'"

Two months later, Brian and his wife introduced David to a young woman of their acquaintance. Twenty-five years old, Jane Fontane was a pretty woman with blue eyes and shoulder-length strawberry blond hair. At five feet one and one hundred and eighty pounds, she was sensitive about her weight, but she carried her generous size easily, and to those who knew her, it seemed merely a natural adjunct to her nurturing personality. When I first met Jane in the summer of 1997, her combination of unflappability, affectionate friendliness, and infectious laughter reminded me of no one so much as the central character in Joyce Cary's comic novel *Herself Surprised*—the unsinkable Sara Monday, the picaresque mother of five children, a woman whom Cary describes as a kind of force of nature, a woman whose earthy goodness and fundamental optimism see her through every scrape life can throw at her—including her own youthful poor judgments.

Like Sara, Jane possessed a guilelessness and innocence that helped to explain how, by the time she met David, she was herself the single mother of three children—by three different fathers. Unworldly to a fault, Jane was a lifelong nonsmoker and nondrinker, a homebody who did not go to bars and didn't approve of "cursing." Her chief flaw was a certain neediness, a result perhaps of her difficult childhood in Winnipeg, where she was raised by her mother and stepfather.

Jane was sixteen when she joined the civilian cadets—an army program offered at her school as an extracurricular activity. There she met Robert, a cadet a few years older than her. "He was the first guy I ever fell in love with," she says. Robert suggested that they leave Winnipeg and move across the country to his hometown of Bancroft, Ontario. To her parents' chagrin, Jane agreed to the plan. The couple stayed with Robert's parents for the summer, then moved on to Quebec, where Jane soon learned that she was pregnant. Robert talked about marriage, but then he started taking off. "He'd go out for cigarettes and he wouldn't come back for six hours," Jane recalls. One day she saw him on the street holding hands with another girl. Shortly after that, she left and returned home to Winnipeg on the train.

Her parents were furious to learn that she was pregnant, but she was jobless and broke and had no choice but to stay with them. Her daughter was born in 1982. Jane was twenty years old. She was an excellent mother, surrounding her daughter with the love that she felt she had never received from her own parents. Jane eventually moved out to a small apartment in the city's West End, where a friend of a friend introduced her to Dean, a handsome, dark-haired young man who worked as a security guard. They started dating, but he was too young to settle down, even when Jane discovered that she was pregnant again. Their daughter was born in 1984. Dean helped out financially when he could, but his visits gradually grew less frequent and finally stopped altogether. With two infants at home, Jane could not work, but eventually she got a job through a government program and started making money. Life was looking up. Then she met a young man who lived across the way. His name was Raymond. "Our apartment block was right across from each other," Jane says. "He said, 'If you ever want to use my washer and dryer . . .'" Jane took him up on this offer, and more besides.

"I'm not proud of it," Jane says. "But I was really looking for love in all the wrong places. I wanted a relationship. I wanted someone to love me." When Raymond learned that Jane was carrying her third child, he told her about his "common-law wife" who happened to be returning soon from British Columbia. "That's how I lost Raymond," Jane says. Her son was born in the early spring of 1988. Jane was at the lowest point in her life.

Three weeks after her son's birth, Jane got a call from her mother. Anne had some news. Lately she had been keeping house for a young woman recuperating from surgery. Anne had mentioned to this woman Jane's difficult situation, saying that she would probably never find someone to marry her now that she was saddled with three children. The woman had mentioned that she knew a young man who might like to meet Jane: he was her brother-in-law, the identical twin of her husband, Brian.

Jane had little hope for this long-shot matchmaking effort,

but she gave the woman a call. Brian's wife told Jane all about David's accident and how he had received a substantial sum of money as a settlement. "She said he's got this *van* and a *convertible*. I said, 'Does it really matter how much money he has or what he has between his legs? If he's not good to me or the kids, he can go his own way.' "

The two women arranged a day when Jane would go to Brian's house and meet David. The two hit it off right away. David, who was probably the more nervous of the two, says, "She had such a true heart."

The foursome made plans for a double date and that weekend went to a restaurant. At the end of the night, David held Jane's hand, and they made a date to meet each other alone. Soon they were dating regularly, and as they fell increasingly for each other, David began to worry about when, and how, to tell Jane about his injury. He finally got up the nerve one day while they were driving in his van up to his cabin in the woods. He had not got more than a few words out when Jane stopped him. She told him she already knew, and she didn't care about it. "She said that she had known all that time and she didn't want to tell me because she figured it would bother me," David recalls. "That's when I knew it was the real thing; I knew that she cared for *me.*"

Asked her feelings about knowing her husband was raised to age fifteen as a girl, Jane treats it as a fact less to be marveled at than one to inspire outrage. "When I saw those pictures of him as Brenda, I just shook my head and thought, Poor child. He didn't look like a girl to me. He looked like Dave. I thought, Going to school must have been the hardest thing."

In the fall of 1989, they moved into an apartment together. David's phalloplasty allowed him to have sex with Jane. "You know how it is when you get into a relationship," Jane laughs. "You do it a lot in the first year."

David sold his "Shaggin' Wagon"—emblem of the reckless, oats-sewing youth that he had never actually had. With the money, he bought a diamond ring.

"I remember," Jane says, "he came into the bedroom and he said, in a very serious voice, 'I want to talk to you.' We were sitting on the bed. He took out this box and opened it up. There was a ring inside. My eyes were like saucers. He said, 'Will you marry me?' "

On 22 September 1990, two years and four months after they first met, David Peter Reimer and Jane Anne Fontane were married at a ceremony in Regents Park United Church in the city of Winnipeg. Jane's two daughters were bridesmaids. David wore a white tuxedo; Jane wore a white dress. Standing before the congregation of some one hundred and thirty guests, made up of friends and family, on an unseasonably warm fall morning, David and Jane spoke the vows that they had written for one another.

"Jane," David said, "I take you to be my wife; to laugh with you in joy, to grieve with you in sorrow, to grow with you in love, to be faithful to you alone, as long as we both shall live."

And Jane said to him, "David, I choose you to be my life's partner. I promise to respect you, to encourage you, to forgive you and instill hope in you. I give you my love for this day, and for all the days to come."

PART THREE

As Nature Made Him

≡

13

=

KEITH SIGMUNDSON REMEMBERS his discomfort on seeing the advertisement. It appeared, he says, sometime in the
1980s in an American Psychiatric Society newsletter, and it
said: "Will whoever is treating the twins please report."
Below this entreaty was a name and address: Dr. Milton Diamond, University of Hawaii-Manoa, John A. Burns School of
Medicine, Honolulu.

"I saw it," Sigmundson says, "but I couldn't bring myself
to answer."

In the ten years that had elapsed since Brenda's switch to
David in 1980, Sigmundson had toyed with the idea of publishing the true outcome of the case. He hadn't done it, and for
a very simple reason. "I was shit-scared of John Money," he
admits. "I didn't know what it would do to my career." It had
been one thing for Sigmundson to cooperate with the BBC
documentary and appear as an unidentified psychiatrist speaking about "difficulties" in the twin's psychological adjustment.

It would be quite another to challenge a man of Money's power directly by publishing a signed article describing how his most widely publicized and influential case had failed from the outset. Sigmundson put the idea out of his head. Diamond's ad was an awkward reminder. At first, Sigmundson almost answered it, but he had resisted the urge.

Money himself also mastered any urge he might have felt to publicize the case's outcome. After his encounter with the BBC reporters in October 1979, he dropped all direct references to the case from his published papers, books, and public lectures. To many in the field of sexual development, his sudden silence on the subject was perplexing.

Virginia Prince, a pioneering transvestite activist who founded the first magazine for cross-dressers, *Transvestia*, in 1960, was one of those curious about the fate of the case, since it had played a significant role in her own acceptance of herself and her sexuality. Born a male, Charles Prince was in his early teens when he first started dressing in women's clothes for erotic gratification—a clandestine activity that continued even after his marriage and the birth of his son. In his forties, Prince began to live full-time in the role of a woman, divorcing his second wife and changing his name to Virginia. Though a fully "out" transvestite by the time she learned of the twins case, Prince says that the story of the sex-changed baby nevertheless had a profound impact on her.

She first learned of it at a meeting of the Society for the Scientific Study of Sex (or Quad-S), an association of sex researchers and activists for which Money served as president for two years in the early 1970s. It was at a November 1972 Quad-S meeting in Palm Springs, California, that then-president Money gave a sneak preview of the twins case—one month before its wider unveiling at the American Association for the Advancement of Science in Washington, D.C.

"John presented pictures of the twins," Prince recalls. "One photograph was of the two kids playing. The girl had a bow in her hair and was wearing a little dress; she's sitting in the front of a wheelbarrow, and her brother is driving her around. The other was a portrait—a snapshot, but it was posed. The little boy's got kind of a scowl on his face, and he's not attempting to make a good showing. But the little girl is sitting up straight and smiling and looking at the camera, just as if she's saying, 'I'm happy as a clam.' That's the picture that got stamped on everybody's mind."

For Prince, Money's twins case was encouraging proof that sex and gender were not an immutably preordained biological phenomenon. At every subsequent meeting with Money, Prince asked for an update on the twins' progress. Ordinarily Money was happy to oblige. "He was very upbeat and happy with the results and proud [of] what was done," says Prince. At a lecture in Los Angeles a decade later, that attitude had changed, Prince recalls. It had been some time since she had heard Money comment on the case, and Diamond's paper on the BBC's investigation was yet to be published. "I asked him, 'Whatever became of the twins?'" Prince says. "He wasn't very forthcoming. He seemed to be a little bit put out that I should ask the question. He was very short about it."

At Johns Hopkins, Money grew similarly tight-lipped about the case. Deflecting questions about the twins when the topic arose on the wards or in his classroom, Money told especially inquisitive students and colleagues that he had "lost track" of the experiment after a "media invasion" by reporters. "He said that this family had been victimized by the BBC," says Money's former student Howard Devore, and that "the family and the case had been irreparably damaged as a result." Money offered a similar explanation for his silence to his protégé, Dr. June Reinisch, a psychologist who had become head of the Kinsey Institute after studying with Money in the 1960s. "[He said] he'd been cut off from the family because they had somehow blamed him for the BBC," Reinisch says.

This interpretation of events does not accord with Janet Reimer's recollections. She says that even after the BBC's visit to Winnipeg, she stayed in touch with Money. "I wrote him a letter about David switching back to being a boy and about what was happening in his life," Janet says. "David had got his [settlement money from the hospital] by then. He was already dating girls—maybe not dating, but hanging out with girls." Janet says that Money wrote back. "He said he would like to hear from David and Ron. And I wrote him a letter stating the truth: 'Ron and David do not wish to communicate with you.' I said, 'I'm telling you that as a friend; I don't want to give you a feeling of rejection, but they just don't want to deal with you.'" Janet says that Money retained a studious neutrality in his letters about the news that Brenda was now David. "He never let on that he was disappointed," Janet says. They continued to exchange letters sporadically through the 1980s. Money wrote to Janet about a trip he had made to Zimbabwe; he informed her of his bout with prostate cancer; and he mentioned the removal of his Psychohormonal Research Unit from the main campus of Johns Hopkins in 1986.

Apparently forgetting this exchange of letters, Money continued to insist to his scientific, academic, and medical colleagues that the case was "lost to follow-up"—a surprising claim if for no other reason than that the Reimers continued to live in the very house that Money had visited in 1979 and with the same telephone number that he had used to contact them.

While Money refrained from mentioning the twins case directly in his public statements after 1980, he continued to lecture on the efficacy of infant sex reassignment for boys with no penis, and Johns Hopkins Hospital continued to perform the procedure, even when an alternative treatment was developed in the mid-1970s by Dr. Mel Grumbach at the University of California, San Francisco, for cases of boys born with small penises. He discovered that he could increase phallus size in babies born with micropenis by giving injections of testosterone to the organ shortly after birth. In patients whose bodies were responsive to the hormone, the penis could be made to grow to a length that permitted standing urination and conventional copulation.

Grumbach spoke about the procedure at the Seventh Annual Birth Defects Institute Symposium on Genetic Mechanisms of Sexual Development, held in November 1976 in Albany, New York. He was surprised to discover that he could not earn an endorsement for the procedure from Johns Hopkins, still the single most influential hospital for intersex treatment. The meeting's chairman, Johns Hopkins pediatric endocrinologist Robert Blizzard (who had worked as a consultant to Money on Bruce Reimer's conversion to Brenda back in 1966), articulated the hospital's decision not to adopt the California team's treatment plan. "I think that we will be able to answer the question concerning the preference of rearing of those with [micropenis] in a few years—although not immediately," Blizzard said in his closing remarks to the symposium. "I believe that Dr. Grumbach's group on the West Coast is going to do what they believe is correct; namely, raise these children as boys; and our group on the East Coast are going to do what they think is correct; namely, raise these children as girls."

John Money was Johns Hopkins's most tireless promoter of that decision in the years that followed, stating in interviews, speeches, books, and papers that sex reassignment to girlhood was the sole option for baby boys with micropenis—or boys who, like David Reimer, had lost their penis to injury. At a meeting of the National Institute of Child Health and Human Development in September 1987, Money mentioned such infant sex changes as being among his most important clinical contributions to medical science. The occasion for Money's comments was a ceremony at which he was being honored as one of four scientists in the country who had, for twenty-five consecutive years, been funded with taxpayers' money by the National Institutes of Health. "In syndromes of male hermaphroditism and micropenis, and in cases of *ablatio penis* from circumcision trauma, when there is insufficient phallic tissue for surgical reconstruction of an adequate urinary and copulatory penis, a baby may be assigned and clinically habituated as a girl," Money told the NIH audience in his acceptance speech. "In adulthood, comparison of such cases with those living as males without a penis shows a higher prevalence of satisfactory outcome in those living as females."

Money's comments were curious for at least two reasons: (1) no systematic follow-up studies had ever been published by Money, or Johns Hopkins, that demonstrated the prevalence of this satisfactory outcome, nor have there been in the years since Money's remarks; and (2) at the time that he described the ability of doctors to successfully change the sex of *developmentally normal boys* to girls in cases of penis loss, the only such experiment he had followed from babyhood to adulthood was that of Brenda Reimer—an experiment that had failed fully seven years earlier, when Brenda had become David.

14

≡

Mɪʟᴛᴏɴ Dɪᴀᴍᴏɴᴅ ѕᴀʏѕ that he cannot recall what spurred his decision to refocus his attention on the twins case at the dawn of the 1990s. He says that he had simply grown impatient with the silence around the experiment. "My thinking at that time was, This person has to be an *adult* now," Diamond says. "We should be able to write an article about this."

Further incentive for returning to the subject was soon provided by Money himself, who in 1991 published *Biographies of Gender and Hermaphroditism in Paired Comparisons*, a career-summing monograph on his forty years of work at the Psychohormonal Research Unit. Presenting his largest collection to date of "matched pairs" the book was Money's latest defense of his theory that social learning overrides biological imperatives in the shaping of human sexual identity. Missing from the text was mention of the definitive test for his thesis—his ultimate matched pair: the sex-changed twin and her brother. In the book's introduction, Money explained the mysterious absence of the case from this otherwise comprehensive volume—an absence that he insinuated owed something to the machinations of his longtime challenger, Milton Diamond.

"On the international academic scene," Money wrote, "doctrinal rivalry regarding the origins of gender identity led to an alliance with an unscrupulous media"—here he inserted a parenthetical reference to Diamond's 1982 paper on the troubled case—"that prematurely terminated a unique longitudinal study of identical twins. A BBC crew of television sleuths, incited by the prospect of airing a doctrinal dispute, traced the whereabouts of the twins and their family and unethically invaded their privacy for programming purposes." Money provided no information about Brenda's 1980 decision to become David, and this brief reference, with its hint that Diamond was somehow connected to the case's premature termination, marked Money's last published comment on the case.

Perhaps understandably, Diamond was disinclined to allow this innuendo-steeped passage to stand as the final historical word on the twins experiment. That the academic community at large accepted Money's version of events was clear from yet another book published that year: *John Money: A Tribute*, a collection of essays written on the occasion of Money's seventieth birthday. Replete with paeans to Money's scholarship from longtime acolytes, including Anke Ehrhardt and June Reinisch, the volume also included a fulsome tribute from Dr. John Bancroft, a psychiatrist and clinical consultant at the Royal Edinburgh Hospital in Scotland, who is now director of the Kinsey Institute. A behaviorist who was a believer in the primacy of rearing over biology in sexual orientation, Bancroft had taken this nurturist view to its logical conclusion in his clinical work. As a sex therapist in Great Britain, he had experimented with trying (in vain) to convert adult homosexuals to heterosexuality through aversion therapy. In his tribute to Money, Bancroft referred with tart disapproval to the "recurring attack from Diamond" and went on to cast doubts on the veracity of the information Diamond had reported from the BBC about the psychological difficulties Brenda had suffered.

"Money has reported her development at various stages, consistent with his theoretical expectations," Bancroft wrote. "However, since the prepubertal stage, the scientific community has received no further authoritative reports, but rather rumors (*not* from Money) of troubled developments." He moved on to defend Money's decade-long silence on the case, casting it as evidence of Money's scrupulous care for the emotional health of his research subjects. "In a case such as this," wrote Bancroft, "when the attention of the scientific community (and in this case the media also) is focused on a particular individual, it is easy to see the need to withdraw and be silent to protect that individual; it must be extremely difficult to be the living test of a controversial theory!"

With his own academic integrity now being questioned, Milton Diamond did not have the luxury of withdrawing and being silent. Since the late 1970s and through the '80s, he had made periodic inquiries (and placed at least one ad) seeking information from endocrinologists and psychiatrists about the case. But now he resolved to redouble his efforts to learn the fate of the twin.

Through the BBC, Diamond found the name of a psychiatrist who had worked on the case—Dr. Doreen Moggey. That spring, he called her.

It had been fourteen years since Moggey terminated therapy with Brenda. She told Diamond that she did not know the final outcome of the experiment. She did, however, offer to give Diamond a phone number for the man who had overseen Brenda's psychiatric treatment: Keith Sigmundson.

"I remember the first words Sigmundson said to me when I called," Diamond recalls with a chuckle. "It was to the effect of 'I was wondering how long it would take for you to get here.'"

By that time Sigmundson was living in Victoria, British Columbia, where he had become head of the province's Division of Child Psychiatry. "Mickey said, 'Keith, we *gotta* do this,'" Sigmundson remembers. At first Sigmundson tried to beg off, but Diamond, he says, "kept on badgering me a little bit."

As someone who had seen firsthand the results of a reportedly successful sex reassignment, Sigmundson was inclined to agree with Diamond's thesis that the procedure of turning baby boys into girls was wrongheaded. Still, Sigmundson had been warned by colleagues that Diamond was a "fanatic" with an ax to grind. Further conversations with Diamond and a reading of his journal articles convinced Sigmundson otherwise. "I came to see that Mickey is a serious researcher and a caring guy who really believed that Money's theory had caused—and was continuing to cause—great harm to children." Sigmundson agreed to contact David Reimer and ask if he would be willing to cooperate with a follow-up article on his life.

"I wasn't sure what it was all about," David says about the call he received that spring from Sigmundson. At that time David had been married for less than a year and wanted nothing more than to put his tortured past behind him. Sigmundson was persistent, however, and David finally agreed to meet Diamond and see what happened.

Diamond flew to Winnipeg to meet David. Over lunch at a local diner, David learned for the first time about his own fame in the medical literature and how the reported success of his case stood as the precedent upon which thousands of sex reassignments had since been performed—and continued to be performed—. "'There are people who are going through what you're going through every day,' " David recalls Diamond telling him, " 'and we're trying to stop that.' "

David was staggered. "I figured I was the only one," he says. "And here Diamond tells me they're doing all these surgeries based on *me*. That's why I decided to cooperate with Mickey." And there was another reason: David sensed in Diamond one of those people whose response to his sufferings was not purely detached and clinical. "When I told him a few things about my life," David says, "I saw that Mickey had tears on his cheeks."

Over the course of the following year, David and his wife and mother recounted to Diamond and Sigmundson the story of David's harrowing journey from boy to girl and back again. Using these interviews plus the detailed clinical records that had accumulated at the Child Guidance Clinic, Diamond set out, as the paper's lead author, to write up the results. He had promised the Reimers anonymity, agreeing to obscure their location, to omit the names of the local physicians, and to refer to David by pseudonym—or rather pseudonyms, since Diamond was faced with the narrative problem of retelling David's double life as both he and she. He settled on the solution of calling David variously Joan (for when he was Brenda) and John (following his switch back to his genetic sex). Only in a conversation with me two years later did Diamond notice that he had bestowed on John/Joan the Christian names of Money's two most important collaborators: Drs. John and Joan Hampson—an act that Diamond assured me was purely unconscious.

Written over the winter of 1994, the paper cast David's life as living proof of precisely the opposite of what Money had said it proved. Citing the Kansas team's classic work from the late 1950s, Diamond wrote that David's case was evidence that gender identity and sexual orientation are largely inborn, a result of prenatal hormone exposure and other genetic influences on the brain and nervous system, which set limits to the degree of cross-gender flexibility that any person can comfortably display. Diamond argued that while nurture may play a role in helping to shape a person's expressed degree of masculinity or femininity, nature is by far the stronger of the two forces in the formation of a person's private inner sense of self as man or woman, boy or girl.

Powerful as the paper was in presenting anecdotal evidence of the neurobiological basis of sexuality, it also served as a clear warning to physicians about the dangers of surgical sex reassignment for all newborns—not just those like David who are born with normal genitals and nervous system. Diamond argued that the procedure was equally misguided for intersexual newborns, since physicians have no way of predicting in which direction the infant's gender identity has differentiated. To change such children surgically into one sex or the other, he argued, was to consign at least half of them to lives as tortured as David's.

Accordingly, Diamond and Sigmundson offered a new set of guidelines for management of babies with ambiguous genitalia. Recognizing that a child must be raised as either a boy or a girl, they recommended that doctors continue to assign a firm sex to the baby—but only in terms of hair length, clothing, and name. Any irreversible surgical intervention, they said, must be delayed until the children were old enough to know, and be able to articulate, which gender they felt closest to. Or as Diamond put it to me, "To rear the child in a consistent gender— but keep away the knife."

Diamond was aware that writing the paper would inevitably raise the specter of a personal vendetta against Money. To minimize this danger, he removed from David's quoted utterances all reference to the famous psychologist. "In fact," Diamond says, "Money's name is only mentioned once.

I didn't want it to be an argument ad hominem. I wanted it to be a theoretical discussion."

Nevertheless it took Diamond and Sigmundson two years to find someone willing to publish their paper.

"We were turned down by all these journals that said it was too controversial," says Sigmundson. "*The New England Journal, The Journal of the American Medical Association.*" The article was finally accepted by the American Medical Association's *Archives of Pediatrics and Adolescent Medicine* in September 1996, with publication set for March 1997. In the intervening months, Diamond and Sigmundson felt considerable apprehension as they waited for their bombshell to go off. "We were basically telling all these physicians that they'd been doing the wrong thing for the past thirty years," Sigmundson says. "We knew we were going to be pissing a lot of people off."

Some critics, as expected, attempted to dismiss the paper on the grounds that Diamond was simply using David's history to embarrass a scientific rival, but at least one physician who saw a prepublication copy of the paper was inclined to agree strongly with its conclusions. Dr. William Reiner had two years earlier launched the first comprehensive long-term follow-up study of patients who had been sex reassigned. Trained as a pediatric urologist, Reiner had actually spent the first eighteen years of his medical career in California performing "normalizing" genital surgeries on intersexual children. It was early in his career that Reiner had his first glimmer of doubt about the Johns Hopkins treatment model. "I got babies and two-year-olds and four-year-olds and eight-year-olds and sixteen-year-olds," he says. "So I really saw a longitudinal view of all these urological conditions—all these birth defects—and I was therefore able to visualize in a relatively short period of time the kinds of effects that these conditions have on the lives of these kids and their families." Then, in 1986, Reiner met a patient who changed his life.

She was a fourteen-year-old girl—a Hmong immigrant— who had announced that she was dropping out of high school because she was "not a girl." To all outward appearances an anatomically normal female, she had nevertheless always rejected girls' play and had insisted on wearing gender-neutral clothes. At puberty she had arrived at the unshakable conviction that she wanted to change sex and live as a male. Referred to Reiner to discuss the possibility of reconstructive surgery, she was threatening suicide unless her wishes were met.

"I had a complete medical workup on the child done," says Reiner. Tests revealed that "she" was biologically a he—a 46XY male who suffered from a rare chromosomal condition that prevents masculine differentiation of the genitals. Reiner performed sex change surgery, after which the former girl effortlessly assumed the sex written in his DNA. The case convinced Reiner of what he had suspected for years: that the biological underpinnings for psychosexual identity are not so easily overridden by social and environmental rearing as he (and every other pediatric urologist, endocrinologist, psychiatrist, and psychologist) had been taught. This further forced Reiner to the uncomfortable conclusion that he had been doing the wrong thing in his surgical career in helping to steer intersexual children into one sex or the other at birth. In a 1996 edition of the *Journal of the American Academy of Child and Adolescent Psychiatry*, Reiner published a paper on the Hmong case, along with a warning to his fellow physicians about the long-accepted theory that rearing prevails over biology in shaping human sexuality.

Reiner also did something else. After eighteen years as a surgeon, he put down his scalpel. He began to retrain as a child psychiatrist specializing in psychosexual development and intersexual conditions. In 1995 he was hired by Johns Hopkins as an assistant professor in psychiatry. There he launched his study on the long-term psychosexual implications of sex reassignment. Reiner set out to follow sixteen patients, focusing particularly on six genetic males who were born without penises and as a result were castrated and raised as girls. Two years into his study, he noted that all six sex-changed boys were closer to males than to females in attitudes and behavior. Two had spontaneously reverted to being boys without being told of their male (XY) chromosome status.

"These are children who did not have penises," Reiner told me, "who had been reared as girls and yet *knew* they were boys. They don't say, 'I wish I was a boy' or 'I'd really rather be a boy' or 'I think I'm a boy.' They say, 'I *am* a boy.'" Reiner stressed the parallels between the children he was studying and David Reimer, who also "knew," despite his rearing as Brenda, that he was not a girl. Reiner wrote a supportive editorial in *Archives of Pediatrics and Adolescent Medicine* to accompany Diamond and Sigmundson's John/Joan paper.

Today Reiner says that both David's case and the trend in his own study support the findings that have emerged on the primacy of neurobiological influences on gender identity and sexual orientation. He cites the now-classic study done at Oxford University in 1971, which showed anatomic differences between the male and female brain in rats. Six years later, at UCLA, researchers narrowed these differences to a cluster of cells in the hypothalamus. A study done in the mid-1980s in Amsterdam located the corresponding area in the human hypothalamus, noting that it is twice as large in homosexual as in heterosexual men. Further studies have supported this finding. In 1993 and again in 1995, researcher Dean Hamer announced that in two separate studies of gay male brothers, he had found a certain distinctive pattern on their X chromosomes. The finding suggested that sexual orientation may have a genetic component.

Although Hamer's studies have failed to be replicated by other scientists, few sex researchers today dispute the mounting evidence of an inborn propensity for acting as, and inwardly identifying with, a particular sex. "It's quite clear that the vast majority of boys born with functioning testicles have masculine brains," Reiner says. He endorses Diamond and Sigmundson's recommendation to delay surgery in cases of penile loss or intersexuality and to impose only a provisional assignment that can be changed should the child voice a strong desire to live as the other sex. Reiner suggests that this treatment model is diametrically opposed to the one pioneered at Johns Hopkins by Money and his colleagues, in which a sexual identity is imposed on a child through unshakable fiat of physicians, and any doubts or confusions the child may express about the assignment are denied by caregivers. Reiner says that on the basis of David's case and the others he has studied, the decades-old Johns Hopkins treatment model needs to be reevaluated. "We have to learn to listen to the children themselves," he says. "They're the ones who are going to tell us what is the right thing to do."

Before Diamond and Sigmundson's journal article appeared in the *Archives of Pediatrics and Adolescent Medicine* in March 1997, the American Medical Association's public relations department alerted the media that something explosive was coming. On the day of the article's publication, the *New York Times* ran a front-page story headlined SEXUAL IDENTITY NOT PLIABLE AFTER ALL, REPORT SAYS, in which writer

Natalie Angier described David's life as having "the force of allegory." Twenty-four years after publishing news of the case's success, *Time* magazine ran a full-page story declaring, "The experts had it all wrong." Similar news accounts appeared around the world—and soon Diamond and Sigmundson were deluged with calls from reporters in several countries seeking an interview with the young man now known simply as John/Joan.

David agreed to appear on two television newsmagazine programs. He was shown in darkened silhouette on ABC-TV's *Primetime Live* and with his face obscured in a Canadian Broadcasting Corporation documentary. It was during the latter taping, which took place in New York City in June 1997, that I was introduced to David by Diamond and Sigmundson. The researchers had passed along to David the names of the many reporters who had requested an interview with him, but David (a rock'n' roll fan) had chosen the reporter from *Rolling Stone*.

At that first meeting with me, David was nervous and guarded. He explained that his childhood had made it difficult for him to trust strangers, but later, over a beer at the Hard Rock Cafe, he grew more relaxed. He spoke about how his parents and brother had been crucial supports in a childhood that he described as "a pit of darkness." I soon learned that a formidable sense of humor had also played a role in his survival. Describing the physical differences between himself and his heavier, slightly balding twin, he shouted over the pounding music, "I'm the young *cool* Elvis. He's the fat *old* Elvis."

But the strongest impression I was left with was of David's unequivocal masculinity. His gestures, walk, attitudes, tastes, vocabulary—none of them betrayed the least hint that he had been raised as a girl. And indeed, when I asked whether he thought his extraordinary childhood had given him a special insight into women, he dismissed the question. David had apparently never *been* a girl—not in his mind, where it counts. He insisted that his conversion from Brenda at age fourteen marked nothing more than a superficial switch in name—as if the double mastectomy, two phalloplasties, and lifelong course of testosterone injections he needs to compensate for his castration were mere details. "I've changed over," David said, "but mainly by name. The rest was all cosmetic. I just had repaired what was damaged. That's all."

Through the summer and fall of 1997, David's story continued to receive media coverage. With this coverage, another set of voices in the debate over the heretofore unexamined practice of infant sex reassignment began to be heard. These were the voices of those intersexes born after the publication of Money's 1955 protocols—people in their thirties and forties who as babies had undergone normalizing genital surgeries and sex assignments and who were now ready to speak on the record about their lives.

They had already begun to emerge as a public voice four years earlier, largely through the efforts of one person: a San Francisco–based activist named Cheryl Chase, who had been lobbying for changes in intersex treatment since the early 1990s. "I wasn't getting very far," admits Chase, a short-haired woman with a dry, rational manner that belies the passion driving her. "That changed overnight when the John/Joan case blew up."

At her birth in suburban New Jersey in 1956, Chase presented a classic case of ambiguous genitalia. Instead of a penis and testicles, there was a somewhat vaginalike opening behind her urethra, and a phallic structure of a size and shape that could be described as either an enlarged clitoris (if she were assigned as a girl) or a micropenis (if a boy). After three days of deliberation, the doctors told Chase's parents that their child should be reared as a boy. She was christened Charlie. But a year and a half later, her parents, still troubled by Charlie's unusual appearance, consulted another team of experts. They reassigned her as a girl and told her parents that she would grow up to be a happy, healthy, normal woman. Her parents changed her name from Charlie to Cheryl, and the doctors removed her clitoris.

Like David Reimer, Chase was then raised without knowledge of her true birth status. Thus, like David, she experienced a childhood punctuated with mysterious, unexplained surgeries and regular genital and rectal exams. Also like David, she grew up confused about her sex. "I was more interested in guns and radios," Chase says, "and if I tried to socialize with any kids, it was generally boys, and I would try to physically best my brother. I didn't fit with boys or girls, I was stigmatized and ostracized by my peers, and picked out for teasing all the time." At age ten, Cheryl's parents brought her to a psychiatrist, who attempted to prepare Cheryl for her role as wife and mother. As a preadolescent, she recognized that she was erotically attracted to females.

By age nineteen, Chase had done some of her own medical sleuthing and understood that she had been subjected to a clitorectomy as a child, and she began to search for her medical history. She was thwarted by her doctors, who refused to reveal the circumstances of her birth. It took three years for her to find a physician willing to disclose her medical records. It was then that Chase read that doctors had labeled her a "true hermaphrodite"—a term that refers to people whose gonads possess both ovarian and testicular tissue. This was also when she first learned that she had spent the first eighteen months of her life as a boy named Charlie, and that her parents, doctors, aunts, uncles, grandparents, and family friends had conspired to keep this secret from her. She also learned that the operation she had undergone at age eight (to relieve "stomachaches") had actually been to cut away the testicular part of her gonads.

Horrified and angered at the deceptions perpetrated upon her and aggrieved at the loss of her clitoris, which had rendered her incapable of orgasm, Chase began to seek out others like herself. Through letters to the editors of medical journals and magazines, news articles, listings with crisis hotlines, and ultimately on a website, she established a network of intersexes in cities across the country. In 1993, she dubbed the group the Intersex Society of North America, a peer support, activist, and advocacy group. By mid-1999, Chase had been contacted by nearly four hundred intersexes from around the world—many of whom told stories almost identical to her own.

To meet Chase and members of ISNA—as I did in the spring of 1997, when they held a peaceful demonstration outside Columbia Presbyterian Hospital in New York, where Chase's clitoral amputation was performed—is to enter a world where it is impossible to think of sex with the binary boy-girl, man-woman distinction we're accustomed to. There was Heidi Walcutt, genetically male with an XY chromosome constitution but born with a rudimentary uterus, fallopian tubes, internal sperm ducts, and a micropenis, who describes herself as a "true American patchwork quilt of gender." There was Martha Coventry, born with an enlarged clitoris but a fully functioning female reproductive system, who is the mother of two girls. There was Kiira Triea, assigned as a boy at age two, who did not learn of her intersexuality until puberty, when she began to menstruate through her phallus. At that stage she was referred as a patient to Dr. Money at the Psychohormonal Research Unit, where she was treated from age fourteen to seventeen, in the mid-1970s, concurrent with Brenda Reimer.

Kiira and David have never met or spoken, but Kiira's

story bears striking parallels to his. She describes how Dr. Money, evidently attempting to ascertain whether she possessed a male or a female gender identity, questioned her about her sex life—in the frank language for which he is well known. "Have you ever fucked somebody?" she remembers Money asking. "Wouldn't you like to fuck somebody?" She also describes how Money showed her a pornographic movie on a projector he kept in his office. "He wanted to know who I identified with in this movie," she says.

Contrary to Money's claim that an intersexual baby reared as a boy will develop an unequivocal male gender identity, Triea's sexuality and sense of self proved to be far more complicated than that. At fourteen she agreed to undergo feminizing surgery at Johns Hopkins to simulate female genitals, but when she became sexually active for the first time at age thirty-two, her erotic orientation was toward women.

The other intersexes in Chase's group show a similarly complex sexuality. Max Beck was first assigned and reared as a girl named Judy. Despite strong masculine thoughts, inclinations, behaviors, and attitudes, Judy tried to stick with her assignment in order to placate worried parents and relatives, even going so far as to marry in her early twenties. But at age twenty-seven Judy left the marriage and divorced. At the age of thirty-two she stopped taking estrogen, changed her name to Max, and began taking testosterone by patch. Yet even today, Max resists the simple designation of male. "I have always felt—and continue to feel myself to be—intersexed," he recently e-mailed me. " 'Masculine' is simply a more comfortable compromise, testosterone a tastier hormonal cocktail than estrogen." Not all the intersexes who joined Chase were sex-reassigned as babies. Dr. Howard Devore, the psychologist who studied under John Money in the 1980s, was born in 1958 with acute hypospadius (a penis open from base to tip) and with undescended, underdeveloped testicles, but was raised as a boy. Beginning at age three months he endured some sixteen "normalizing" surgeries through childhood, aimed at giving him a cosmetically convincing penis. The experience, Devore says, was emotionally devastating—and wholly unnecessary. His genitals still do not resemble those of a normal male and the sole result of his constant hospitalizations is a psychological scarring far worse than he would have experienced had he been raised with counseling to accept his atypical genitals. Devore refrained from making this argument to Money. "I learned very early that if you choose to do battle with John," he says, "you have to deal with a very, very angry man who's going to make you feel horrible for challenging him." (Devore says that only in the wake of the "John/Joan" revelations has he felt emboldened to make his intersexuality public—and to openly challenge his former professor.)

Armed with her own story and those of her fellow intersexes, Chase began trying to alert the medical establishment to the dangers of the protocols for intersex management initiated by Johns Hopkins. ISNA's stated aim was to abolish all cosmetic genital surgery on infants—not simply the castration and sex reversal of micropenis boys. While Chase did not oppose life-saving corrective surgery on genitals, she denounced as "barbaric" all medically unnecessary cosmetic treatments on newborns that could have an irreversible effect on their erotic or reproductive functioning. And ultimately, she said, she wanted to "end the idea that it's monstrous to be different."

Chase found it more difficult than she had anticipated to gain an audience with influential people in the field—including John Money. "I've written him several times, politely, asking if he would clarify his position for us," Chase told me. "Each time he would return my letters with a note scribbled on the corner saying he doesn't have enough time to talk to me."

Chase also wrote to the American Academy of Pediatrics—an association with a membership of over fifty-five thousand doctors in the United States, Canada, and Latin America. The AAP has long endorsed Money's protocols for intersex treatment. "I write to inform you that many who have been treated according to the model you outline have found that the treatment itself has rendered our lives an ordeal," Chase wrote to the AAP in 1995. "We who are intersexual have been discussing our experiences through the Intersex Society of North America . . . and we find that the current model of treatment does nothing to discourage the shame and secrecy surrounding intersexuality. . . . We would love to open a dialog with you, and we encourage you to mention, when you teach about treatment of intersex, the existence of a vocal, organized population of intersexual former patients who oppose the current model."

The AAP did not respond to this letter. Chase wrote to them again in 1996 and again received no response. That October, Chase and other ISNA members held a demonstration at the AAP's national conference in Boston. Academy officials refused to meet with the protesters, but they did distribute a press release among the journalists and protestors at the demonstration. "The American Academy of Pediatrics, a voice for children for over 60 years, is aware of the concerns and sensitive to the needs of intersexuals," the statement read. It went on to say that the AAP would not change its stance on intersex treatment and cited Money's work from the 1950s to defend its position.

Chase also appealed to former Surgeon General Joycelyn Elders, who prior to her appointment to Clinton's administration had practiced for over twenty years as a pediatric endocrinologist in Arkansas, where she regularly applied Money's protocols for intersex management to ambiguously sexed new-borns. Elders never acknowledged Chase's letters.

In 1996, Chase did succeed in persuading the *New York Times* to write a feature article about the burgeoning intersex activist movement, but in the story members of the medical establishment refused to discuss ISNA's complaints. Dr. John Gearhart, head of pediatric urology at Johns Hopkins, dismissed the group as "zealots." In a conversation with me in the summer of 1997, amid the media storm generated by Diamond and Sigmundson's article on the failed twins case, Gearhart was more politic when addressing the issues raised by ISNA and David's case. While he insisted that sex reassignment remains a viable option for boys born with micropenis or who lose their penises to injury, he noted that advances in penile reconstruction made him more hesitant to recommend the procedure today. "If John/Joan happened today," he told me, "I would sit down with those parents and say, 'The child has testicles; it's a normal male child.' I would suggest that you *could* change the child's gender, but I would not recommend that, because reconstructive genital surgery has come light-years since John/Joan's accident."

Gearhart also said that advances in medicine render ISNA's concerns obsolete. "When these people in ISNA were operated on, twenty-five and thirty years ago, there weren't really children's reconstructive surgeons around," he said. "So most of [these babies] had their clitoris or their penis amputated. That was wrong, OK? *That* was wrong. But the surgeons didn't know any better. Nowadays, people in modern reconstructive surgery are not cutting off little babies' clitorises or penises, or anything along those lines." Gearhart said that modern micro-surgery retains sensation.

To hear the back-and-forth exchanges of doctors like Gearhart and activists like Cheryl Chase is to be convinced that the issues involved will not be settled anytime soon. For instance, Chase flatly rejects Gearhart's claim that surgeons maintain clitoral sensation after reducing the organ's size. Gearhart meanwhile continues to reject ISNA's call for change in the current treatment protocols, insisting that scores of intersexes live happily in the sex assigned to them in infancy and that Chase and the members of ISNA represent only the "disgruntled" few—a charge to which Chase and other ISNA members take particular exception. They insist that silence among intersexual adults does not reflect happiness with the decisions made for them as babies, but is instead a symptom of the shame and secrecy that are the legacy of the current treatment methods.

"It goes back to being completely isolated as children," Heidi Walcutt told me. "*Knowing* that there's this difference, but being silenced and being shamed about it. Some people never get to the point where they start looking for answers—let alone step out as an activist against what was done to them." Chase adds that there is also a strong disincentive for intersexes to speak out, since doing so often means undergoing a traumatic confrontation with parents who authorized the surgeries in the first place. Chase points out that more than a few ISNA members find themselves estranged from their families.

It is obviously difficult for an independent investigator to verify either Gearhart's or ISNA's conflicting claims about the relative happiness of adult intersexes who decline to speak about their lives; they are by definition invisible. Asked to provide a satisfied patient, every pediatric specialist I contacted voiced the Catch-22 that they "lose track" of their patients after young adulthood. Gearhart added, "And the ones I do know just want to live their lives in privacy."

I was able to locate and speak to one intersex who is not a member of ISNA or any other activist group. She is notable in her own right in that in the late 1970s she was repeatedly cited as a particularly successful example of an intersex who was sexually reassigned in infancy. Her case was featured not only on an Emmy-winning ABC-TV science series documentary, but also in the BBC's investigative report on the twins case. She is Paula, the former John Money patient whom Peter Williams and Martin Smith included for balance in their twins case exposé. Living anonymously now in the Northeast, but located through an Internet search engine that lists census records, Paula agreed to speak with me on the condition that I not use her last name or otherwise reveal her identity.

In a series of phone conversations and a five-hour in-person interview with Paula and her mother, I learned the circumstances of Paula's birth. They were in many respects strikingly similar to the stories I had already heard from Chase and her colleagues in ISNA. Born in September 1971, the second of three children, Paula presented ambiguous genitalia with a scrotum but no testicles inside and a small penis of mostly empty skin. The local doctors recommended assignment as a boy, saying that the penis would grow and that the testicles would descend over time. The baby was duly christened Michael Edward. But Michael's mother remained upset by her baby's appearance and continued to consult doctors over the first year and a half of her child's life. When Michael was eighteen months old, a neighbor in whom Michael's mother had confided the dilemma brought over the current issue of *Time* magazine, which carried a story about one of a pair of twin baby boys who had lost his penis to circumcision and was later turned into a girl on the advice of Johns Hopkins psychologist John Money. According to the *Time* article, the sex change had been a complete success. Michael's mother immediately wrote to Dr. Money, who replied promptly and advised that she bring Michael to Baltimore for immediate sex reassignment as a girl.

"Within two days," Paula's mother says, "I was on my way down there with my husband and my child."

On 23 February 1973, Michael was operated on at Johns Hopkins by Dr. Howard Jones, who established that the baby (like Cheryl Chase) had gonads containing both ovarian and testicular cells. Jones removed the undescended gonads (to prevent spontaneous masculinization at puberty) and reconstructed the external genitalia so that they would appear more feminine. Full excavation of a vaginal canal was to wait until the baby was in her teens. In the meantime it was arranged that Paula would return periodically to Johns Hopkins for counseling with Dr. Money. And indeed, Paula's mother brought her daughter back to see Dr. Money several times a year throughout her childhood. Since Dr. Money had often said that Paula was one of his best patients, it came as little surprise to Paula's mother when, shortly after her daughter's seventh birthday, Dr. Money asked if she would be willing to put Paula on television to discuss her successful sex reassignment. "I said, 'If it would help one other person,' " Paula's mother recalls, " 'then that's all I want from it.' "

The program was part of the ABC-TV science series *The Body Human*. The episode, entitled "The Sexes," featured a scene of Paula, a freckle-faced, short-haired girl, during one of her trips to the Psychohormonal Research Unit. With the camera keeping a studious distance from the fertility sculptures arrayed around Money's plant-festooned office, the famous psychologist was shown sitting at his desk, in shirtsleeves and tie. He asked Paula questions as she faced him from a large, afghan-covered armchair. In a flowered dress with lace collar, her fingernails painted bright red, Paula smiled warily as she haltingly answered Money's questions about marriage and career. Meanwhile the narrator explained in voice-over, "At the

Johns Hopkins Hospital, under the enlightened care of specialist Dr. John Money, careful attention is paid to nurturing Paula's image of herself as a girl, preparing her for all the complete experiences of womanhood."

Shortly after this program aired in May 1979, Money again asked Paula's mother to put her daughter in front of the cameras. This time the reporters were with the BBC. Again Paula's mother agreed, and Dr. Money made the preliminary arrangements with Williams and Smith to interview Paula's mother. The filming took place in early October 1979. According to Paula's mother this interview proved less gratifying than her encounter with the ABC-TV producers. Within hours of doing the interview, she received an agitated call from Dr. Money, who told her he had learned that the BBC reporters had an "ulterior motive" in making their documentary. Money wanted Paula's mother to pull out of the interview. When he learned that the reporters had already done the interview, he was irate. "He was absolutely furious with those reporters," she recalls. "*Furious.*" The imbroglio did nothing to mar the relationship between Dr. Money and Paula's mother. She continued to bring her daughter to see Money for regular follow-up visits until Paula was eighteen years old, at which point Paula underwent the final stage of vaginal surgery and stopped going to Johns Hopkins.

Today, at twenty-seven, Paula is a slim woman with blue eyes and tawny, straight, side-parted hair that falls to her waist. Dressed in jeans, a blue shirt, and platform open-toed sandals, she passes easily as a woman, albeit a boyishly figured one. Her small breasts and hip shape are maintained only through a regular lifelong regimen of estrogen ingestion. She takes care to pitch her raspy voice in the upper part of its register, but it does at times dip into lower notes than would ordinarily be expected in even a deep-voiced woman. Paula takes assiduous care of her grooming, lavishing great attention on her long mane of hair;

she pays once-weekly visits to the pedicurist and manicurist for the maintenance of her nails; and in the course of our conversation, she frequently refreshed her makeup with the skill of a trained cosmetician.

Despite these obvious outward efforts to enhance her public femininity, Paula says that privately she has no choice but to think about her medical condition every day. Like the other intersexes I spoke with, Paula's surgically created vagina is a daily reminder that she was not born a typical woman. "I don't look like everyone else does," she says. "Not at all. So of course you're always going to have a constant reminder." Asked if her vagina carries sensation, Paula drags on her cigarette. "There's always lack of sensation where there's scarring," she says. Given these realities, it comes as little surprise to hear Paula say that despite the best efforts of medical science, she has a constant sense of living "with a secret." Asked if there are any close friends to whom she has felt comfortable divulging her secret, Paula's face hardens and she chuckles with brittle cynicism. "You have very few friends in this world—trust me." She takes another drag on her cigarette. "Yeah," she continues in the same tone. "That *anyone* can trust. There are very few people in this world." She says that she had a boyfriend for six years in her late teens and early twenties in whom she confided her secret, and he was understanding. Since then, however, she has preferred to keep her condition, and the circumstances of her birth, to herself.

A virgin at age twenty-seven, Paula says that she has never felt any sexual attraction to women. When I asked about this, she cut me off before I had even finished the question. "Not at all," she said. "Never. Never, at all. Not at all." I asked if, while growing up, she had ever thought, "Maybe I'm a boy," but again she spoke before I could get the question out. "Never," she said. "Never at all."

Paula is open about her desire not to upset her mother by voicing doubts about the decisions made on her behalf as a baby. She insists that she is happy with the choice made to reassign her as a girl—or rather, she expresses the view that no other decision could have been made at the time. "I can't see things being any other way," she tells me. "You know?" She pauses, then resumes. "As far as anybody was concerned at the time, this was, like, the only way."

Like the other former research subjects of John Money to whom I spoke, Paula has vivid memories of her counseling sessions with him. She was shown pictures of men and women engaged in sexual intercourse and queried about the most private aspects of her inner self. "He asked questions that a six-, seven-, nine-, *ten*-year-old would not *ever* be asked," Paula recalls: about masturbation, her private sex fantasies, how to deflect lesbian advances from other girls. "He would *press* you for answers," Paula says. "He would sit there and *press* you and *press* you and *press* you. It was way too much for a child. I always said to my mother, 'I don't know why the hell I have to go to him.' "

Appearing on network television as the world's first openly intersexual seven-year-old was also, Paula says, "traumatic." When she discusses this aspect of her dealings with Dr. Money, Paula's vocabulary and tone of voice lose their quality of studious feminine poise. Her voice drops several tones lower as she spits out a stream of angry expletives. "All that TV bullshit was garbage," she snarled. "It was *bullshit*, it was traumatic. I mean you have to understand, at that time of my life I was in *grade* school. People in my class were asking me about it the next day. I was too young to make my own decisions, but if I had had the choice I never would have done it. But that's my mama," she adds with a forgiving but exasperated smile. "She loves John

Money. She would do anything he said. She thought she was doing good. Helping other mothers. But I think it was bullshit."

Paula's mother has never questioned the decisions she made on Paula's behalf, nor has she questioned John Money's handling of the case. To this day she refers to Money as her "savior" and speaks in only the most glowing terms about him and about her former son's conversion to girlhood. "Everything worked out fantastic with Paula," she told me, speaking in ecstatically upbeat tones in a phone conversation before I met her daughter. "She is full of life and full of fun. She has never confided in me of any worries. She's a character! A real party girl. Loves life, parties, going out, oodles and oodles of friends. The phone never stops." She described Paula as the very quintessence of femininity. "*Loves* being a girl. Loves to shop. Buys the most expensive clothes. And jewelry. Everything is top designer." She said that Paula had never seemed even slightly tomboyish as a child (an observation in contrast to the recollections of one of the ABC-TV producers, whose impression of the seven-year-old Paula was "That little boy stayed a little boy, no matter *what* they did to him").

Paula's mother does voice one small concern about Paula's life today: her daughter's single status. When Paula's parents brought her to Johns Hopkins, Dr. Money had specifically explained that sex reassignment was being done to ensure that Paula could one day marry, have a normal heterosexual love life, and have children by adoption. "Dr. Money looked that far ahead," Paula's mother marvels. Marriage is the one area where Dr. Money's prognostications have yet failed to materialize, but Paula's mother has not given up hope. "For me," she says, "closure will come when Paula gets married." Paula, watching as her mother speaks, takes a hard drag on her cigarette, then looks away.

Paula is dubious that she will ever marry. For one thing there is the delicate circumstance of her unusual genitals—which Paula feels is a severe stumbling block to physical and emotional intimacy with a partner. There is also the fact that Paula views marriage as an outdated institution. So for now, she continues to live at home with her parents. Her father, who suffers from severe clinical depression, confines himself mostly to his room. Most of Paula's dealings are with her mother. It is a close but emotionally complex relationship in which Paula is totally devoted to her mother, despite Paula's spates of brittle snappishness. Having heard many times during the course of her growing up about the severe trauma her birth caused her mother, Paula lives a life dedicated to minimizing any further emotional upset or unease that her existence might cause. Paula has thus told her mother that she will live at home forever to look after her and will "never leave her."

In the meantime Paula devotes herself to her work. Her choice of career, while not unchallenging, does not reflect her extraordinary intelligence. Tested at Johns Hopkins at age ten, Paula's IQ was 132, placing her in the top 2.2 percent of the population. At the time, Money's associate Gregory K. Lehne wrote in Paula's file that her "future academic planning can include college and professional training, with every expectation of success." And in fact Paula had once planned to become a lawyer. She set those ambitions aside in her junior year of college, after her mother mentioned her wish that Paula pursue nursing. Though Paula had always expressed an understandable aversion to all aspects of the medical profession, she nevertheless quit college and enrolled in nursing school. Currently Paula is a registered nurse and is working toward her master's in nursing. Her mother is "ecstatic" about these developments and boasts of how Paula "has not looked back since."

Paula seems to be a young woman determined not to look back. She says that she has no criticism of those intersex activists who are lobbying the medical profession for change, but she takes the position, for herself, that it is better just to get on with life and not stir up the past. When her mother left the house, Paula admitted quietly, "Maybe they *should* wait and give kids the choice about surgery." That, however, is an opinion she is unlikely to pass on to the medical profession. She has turned down a recent request from Johns Hopkins to participate in a follow-up study on sex reassigned patients. She simply does not want to relive her childhood—which she nevertheless insists was a perfectly happy one. But that some degree of unresolved emotion around her childhood might linger is perhaps suggested by the fact that Paula chose obstetrics and gynecology as her nursing specialty. Today she helps to deliver babies in the same small hospital where she was born twenty-seven years ago, as Michael Edward.

The medical establishment's refusal to listen to those intersexes who *have* elected to speak about their experiences is no surprise to Cheryl Chase. "Our position implies that they have—unwittingly at best, and through willful denial at worst—spent their careers inflicting a profound harm from which their patients will never fully recover," Chase once wrote. She says that she does not expect the medical establishment to change its practices unless forced. Chase plans to force them. "I think a context will open up for surgeons who keep doing this to be vulnerable to lawsuits," she told me. "But it's going to take a while to create that context. Right now we can't sue because it's standard practice, and parents give permission. The first thing we want to have happen is that when they make their recommendation to parents, they tell them it's experimental and there's no evidence that it works and that there's plenty of people who've had it done to them who are mad as hell."

There are other needs as well. Anne Fausto-Sterling, an embryologist at Brown University, says that the medical establishment will have to provide education and emotional support to help parents with the difficult task of raising an infant whose genitals are atypical. "At the moment there is no ongoing counseling done by people skilled in psychosexual development," Fausto-Sterling says. "If there was really a wholesale change in this, the medical profession would have to do something like what they've done with genetic counseling—which is to develop a specialty of people who would work with these families long term and help them resolve both emotional and practical questions. The practical questions are very real: What do I do when it comes to undressing in gym? How do I intervene with the school system? There's a different infrastructure that needs to be built and put into place. I think it's the responsibility of the medical profession to do it."

Perhaps the biggest change that will have to take place is in the medical profession's current view of what it means to be reared with ambiguous genitals, since the Money and Hopkins guidelines are predicated on the belief that such a childhood would be psychologically and psychosexually devastating. Studies that would prove the truth of this intuitive observation are hard to come by; case histories of children reared with ambiguous genitals are rare because so few intersexual newborns have avoided surgical intervention. In 1989 a study did appear in the *Journal of Urology* on the lives of twenty males with micropenis who were reared in their biologic sex. Drs. Justine Reilly and C. R. J. Woodhouse of St. Peter's Hospital and The Hospital for Sick Children in London described how these patients, who ranged in age from ten to forty-three years, had all formed healthy male gender identities and "participated in normal male activities in childhood and adolescence." They also reported that nine (75 percent) of the older patients were sexually active and that "vaginal penetration usually is possible but adjustment of position or technique may be necessary." The researchers drew two main conclusions: "A small penis does not preclude normal male role and a micropenis or microphallus alone should not dictate a female gender assignment in infancy."

Reilly and Woodhouse's study, however, looked at the lives of only twenty patients, all of whom had the same syndrome. A much more exhaustive study exists on the lives of untreated intersexes who display a much wider range of conditions than micropenis alone. Written before the advent of the 1955 protocols, it is a unique and fascinating monograph that reviews over two hundred and fifty cases of intersexes who received no surgical intervention as babies. Furthermore, the study directly addresses the question of how children fare when they grow up with genitals of the sex opposite to that in which they are reared. "Do [these people], with such manifest sexual problems to contend with, break down under the strain, as psychiatric theory may lead one to believe," asked the study's author, "or do they make an adequate adjustment to the demands of life?"

Far from manifesting psychological traumas and mental illnesses, the study showed, the majority of patients rose above their genital handicap and not only made an "adequate adjustment" to life, but lived in a way virtually indistinguishable from people without genital difference—a result that clearly amazed the study's author.

"One would not have been surprised had the paradox of hermaphroditism been a fertile source of psychosis and neurosis," the investigator noted. "The evidence, however, shows that the incidence of the so-called functional psychoses in the most ambisexual of the hermaphrodites—those who could not help but be aware that they were sexually equivocal—was extraordinarily low. The incidence of neurotic psychopathology of the classic types, sufficiently severe and incapacitating to be unmistakable, was also conspicuously low." The study pointed out that genital ambiguity led to a "disheartenment" of mood in some patients and a social "reticence" in others but went on to say of these individuals, "there was no evidence that their disheartenment or reticence ordinarily accumulated to the proportions of psychopathology, seriously impairing their ability to cope with the essential business of life"—such as completing their education, going to the office each day, and earning a living each week.

Of particular interest are the study's in-depth interviews with ten intersexes who received no surgery or hormone treatments until they were old enough to make their own decision. Their lives only strengthened the investigator's impression that the condition of the genitalia plays a strikingly insignificant part in the way a person develops a stable and healthy gender identity, not to mention a secure and confident self-image. One patient with an enlarged clitoris at birth did not have the organ surgically reduced until the age of twelve, yet her childhood with masculinized genitalia left no wound on her psyche and did not impair her sense of herself as a girl. "[O]ne appreciates her remarkable stamina and the self-reliant way in which she had consolidated it," the author noted. A second girl with a similar medical history demonstrated a marked "social deftness and complete poise" and, despite her mother's depressions, "had emerged more stable than her adult sister or brother." About another girl whose masculinized genitals were not surgically altered until she consented to it at age twelve, "one would not be justified in saying that she is different from scores of other adolescents." A boy with an untreated micropenis had married at age twenty-four and, the study reported, "is meeting life most successfully without any suspicion of psychopathology. . . . His life is an eloquent and incisive testimony to the stamina of human personality." A "true hermaphrodite" with a micropenis, split scrotum, and breasts at puberty lived as a male with no surgery to correct these anomalies. "The youth is another living testimony . . . to the stamina of human personality in the face of sexual ambiguity of no mean proportions." A seventeen-year-old boy whose micropenis went untreated through childhood and adolescence "is making a stalwart and almost heroic adjustment to life." Likewise, a twenty-year-old born with a small, hypospadic penis that required him to sit to urinate and that went uncorrected until age nineteen; this patient "was almost a model of what the average citizen believes a healthy, well-adjusted American youth should be," the author noted: "confident, self-reliant, and optimistic."

Unfortunately, no experts in the debate on intersex treatment—including Milton Diamond, Bill Reiner, Anne Fausto-Sterling, or Cheryl Chase—has ever made reference to this valuable report. That such a rare and unique study has been overlooked is perhaps not surprising. Never commercially published or distributed, it can be obtained only through written application to the Widener Library at Harvard University, where it was submitted as a senior dissertation to the college's Ph.D. program in 1951. The author was a thirty-year-old doctoral candidate named John Money.

15

≡

John Money has never explained the shift that occurred in his thinking between the time he finished his Harvard thesis and the time he wrote his first papers on intersexes four years later, and he has never publicly commented on any aspect of his work since the revelations in Diamond and Sigmundson's paper.

Now seventy-eight years old and in semiretirement, he has nevertheless remained a prolific and opinionated writer on the subject of sex and sexuality. His latest book, *Unspeakable Monsters*, was published in the spring of 1999. Through the last two decades, his books and articles have continued to appear with regularity, and in the late 1980s he enjoyed an intense courting by the media over the publication of his book *Lovemaps*—Money's term for an individual's particular constellation of erotic tastes and impulses. Profiles and interviews with Money appeared in *Playboy, Cosmopolitan, Psychology Today, Omni,* and the *Atlantic Monthly.* In *Rolling Stone*'s

1990 "Hot Issue," Money was celebrated as the "Hot Love Doctor," and he appeared on various TV programs.

Meanwhile Money was negotiating a subtle shift from his earlier extreme position on the primacy of rearing over biology in the making of boys and girls. In a May 1988 magazine profile, he seemed at some pains to characterize himself as a longtime champion of the role of *biology* in psychological sex differentiation, saying that when he was publishing papers on the behavioral influence of prenatal sex hormones in the 1950s, "many people in various branches of the social sciences were just enraged at the idea that hormones in the bloodstream before you were born could have a sex differentiating influence on you." In the same article, however, Money reiterated his claim that infant boys can, with surgery and hormone treatments, be turned into heterosexual women.

If the last two decades have seen the consolidation of Money's international reputation as one of the single most influential sexologists of the twentieth century, his career at Johns Hopkins has not been without its setbacks. The seeds for Money's problems were sown as early as 1975, when Dr. Joel Elkes, chairman of the Psychiatry Department and Money's longtime protector within the institution, was replaced by Dr. Paul McHugh.

By almost any measure, McHugh, a practicing Catholic and a sworn enemy of all fashions and fads in psychiatry, was John Money's diametrical opposite—save for the forcefulness of his opinions and his determination to put them into action. Today McHugh is famed as psychiatry's most outspoken scourge. In referring to McHugh's "ceaseless campaign to restore sanity to his own profession," a 1997 *Baltimore Sun* profile dubbed him "Dr. Iconoclast" and listed his "annihilating opinions on everything from doctor-assisted suicide (utterly wrong) to multiple personality disorder (it doesn't exist)." The profile also highlighted his excoriating disdain for "dubious practices—and practitioners—in the medical profession," including Dr. Jack Kevorkian, whom McHugh was quoted as calling "insane," and Dr. Bruno Bettelheim, the famous expert on children, whom McHugh called "a habitual liar, thankless friend, vicious bully, and brazen plagiarist."

McHugh has always reserved special scorn for the practice of sex-change surgery on adult transexuals. Classifying transexualism as merely one symptom in a larger complex of personality disorders, McHugh had long believed that psychiatrists should treat such patients with the talking cure, not radical, irreversible surgeries. In a 1992 article in the *American Scholar*, McHugh lambasted transexual surgery as "the most radical therapy ever encouraged by twentieth century psychiatrists" and likened its popularity to the once widespread practice of frontal lobotomy. "Johns Hopkins was one of the places in the United States where [transexual surgery] was given its start," McHugh pointed out in this article. "It was part of my intention, when I arrived in Baltimore in 1975, to help end it."

Two years after McHugh arrived at Johns Hopkins, Dr. Jon Meyer, a Hopkins psychiatrist and former director of the Gender Identity Clinic, produced a long-term follow-up of fifty postoperative and preoperative adult transexuals treated at Johns Hopkins since the clinic was founded in 1966. Meyer reported that none showed any measurable improvement in their lives and concluded that "sex reassignment surgery confers no objective advantage in terms of social rehabilitation." Presented at the American Psychiatric Association's Annual Convention in May 1977, the paper was published two years later in the *Archives of General Psychiatry*. The transgendered community reacted with outrage to the paper's alleged nonscientific methods and aims. To no avail. Its publication was heralded by an October 1979 press conference at Johns Hopkins, where it was announced to the assembled reporters that the Gender Identity Clinic was now closed. John Money was not notified about the press conference and was not consulted about the clinic's closing—an ignominious position for the man who had—virtually single-handed—spearheaded the movement to open it.

McHugh's tenure at Johns Hopkins also coincided with a sudden dramatic erosion in Money's once secure status as the institution's resident sexual revolutionary. In 1983, Money was informed that his controversial evening course in human sexology was being summarily dropped. Three years later, when Money turned sixty-five, he was notified that he would not be allowed to keep his Johns Hopkins office space—a privilege conferred upon some other retirement-age professors—but must remove himself from the campus. He was relocated to a shabby medical arts building four blocks from the hospital and university, across from an empty lot where the local homeless and addicts congregate. There, Money installed himself in one of the building's low-ceilinged basement offices. With a staff now reduced to a single graduate student, Money affixed to the cheap plywood door of his new space the sign he had removed from his former office door. It reads: Johns Hopkins Psycho-hormonal Research Unit.

Even after his physical removal from the institution, Money's problems with Johns Hopkins were not over. In the early 1990s one of his former research subjects raised a complaint against him and against Johns Hopkins. This patient, who wishes to remain anonymous, has asked me to refer to him as "Charlie Gordon"—a pseudonym that he did not choose randomly. It is the name of the protagonist in the 1960s Daniel Keyes novel *Flowers for Algernon*, which was later turned into the Cliff Robertson movie *Charly*. The fictional story of a retarded man who, as an experimental research subject, was turned into a genius, *Charly* bears striking parallels to the life of the man I have agreed to call Charlie Gordon.

Born in 1947, Gordon showed early signs of hypothyroidism, a congenital endocrine disorder whose symptoms include severely stunted growth and retarded intellectual development—syndromes then classified as the condition "cretinism." At age two, Gordon was referred to Lawson Wilkins's pediatric endocrine clinic at Johns Hopkins where he underwent experimental treatments of hormone replacement by ingesting cow thyroid glands in pill form. The treatment increased not only his physical stature, but also his intellectual powers. At age five he became a psychological research subject in the newly created Psychohormonal Research Unit, where John Money would, for the next twenty-five years, conduct adjunct studies on Gordon's adaptation to his changing bodily and intellectual stature. In an article published in the *Journal of Pediatrics* in September 1978, Money singled out Gordon as having demonstrated the largest increase in intelligence of all the research subjects. According to Money, he had gone from an IQ of 84 at age five to an IQ of 127 in adulthood: a 43-point gain that had taken him from low average to superior range—what Money called "a remarkable upgrading."

Over the course of their association, Gordon became one of Money's favorite research subjects and agreed to Money's request that he appear at medical school grand rounds, in which he was studied by scores of Johns Hopkins student doctors. At the same time, Gordon was making regular annual visits to the clinic for in-depth interviews with Money. Gordon found the encounters unsettling. "He was always saying 'fuck,' all the time," Gordon recalls. " 'Fuck this,' and 'fuck that.' As a kid I was raised in somewhat a religious background. When I'd do church things, he'd say, 'Oh, what do you do that shit for?' "

Money also questioned Gordon closely about sex. Believing that Dr. Money's interest in his erotic life was intended to help him cope with the difficulties associated with his condition, Gordon opened up without reserve, detailing the content of his sexual fantasies, describing his masturbation techniques, and recounting his experimental forays into ménage à trois and his childhood experiences of "playing doctor" with a neighborhood girl. Later, in his twenties, Gordon confessed to the insecurities that had gone along with his small stature, admitting that he had once sought relationships with girls many years his junior—some as young as fourteen. Only several years after he stopped treatment with Money did Gordon learn that Money's interest in his sex life was not simply therapeutic in nature.

This realization was brought home to him with particular force on a day in December 1989 when he was browsing in a bookstore and happened upon a copy of Money's latest volume, *Vandalized Lovemaps*. The book detailed Money's theory of how people develop sexual fetishes, perversions, and disorders, and it featured a number of case histories. The first one, entitled "Pedophilia in a Male with a History of Hypothyroidism," caught Gordon's eye. He began to scan the opening sentences and realized with amazement and horror that the case history being detailed was his own. He saw his sexual life laid out with extensive verbatim quotations culled from his taped interviews with Money and saw himself diagnosed as a pedophile on the evidence of his interest in teenage girls. More shocking still, says Gordon, was information published about his parents, which included a statement by Gordon's father, who had allegedly told Money that Gordon's mother had had an incestuous affair with her brother. Though Gordon and his family were not mentioned by name, he felt that the details of the case would be unmistakable to anyone who knew him or his family. Stricken, Gordon phoned Money, but he could not reach him. "He wouldn't return my calls," Gordon says. "His associate said, 'He's busy.' "

In the spring of 1990, Gordon brought a formal complaint against Money and Johns Hopkins through the federal Department of Health and Human Services Office for Protection from Research Risks—a division of the National Institutes of Health. Gordon learned that scientists operating under federal research grants must adhere to stringent rules, which include gaining informed, signed consent from patients and research subjects about whom a researcher wishes to publish. Money had never secured consent from Gordon for the publication of the deeply private material in *Vandalized Lovemaps*. The Department of Health and Human Services launched an investigation and concluded that "given the nature of [the] information [disclosed by Money], the complainant could be indentifiable by persons acquainted with [him]." That fall, DHHS cited the Johns Hopkins University School of Medicine for "serious non-compliance" with federal regulations for the protection of human research subjects. Calling for "strong corrective action," DHHS required that the Johns Hopkins Psychiatry Department "republish departmental guidelines for safeguarding the identity of patients" and allow patients who did provide informed consent to review manuscripts before publication, and it demanded that Gordon receive an apology from Money in person and in the presence of his department chairperson, in this case Money's nemesis, Dr. Paul McHugh. Gordon says that this apology was never given, but he felt vindicated by the other sanctions. In a statement that Gordon prepared for an October 1997 meeting of President Clinton's National Bioethics Advisory Commission on human research subjects, he outlined his unhappy history with Dr. John Money and drew a parallel between his experiences as a research subject and those of the famous "John/Joan" whose story had broken in the press just eight months earlier.

Despite this string of professional reversals, embarrassments, and punishments, Money remained defiant, combative, and uncowed. Indeed the setbacks seemed only to fuel his contentious spirit. Increasingly his published work appeared to be as much an opportunity for Money to settle scores and air grievances as it was to elucidate the subject of human sexuality. His preface to the 1987 book *Gay, Straight and In Between,* a volume ostensibly about the origins of sexual orientation, included an unusual digression into his then-recent ouster from Johns Hopkins. "In the spring of 1986," he wrote, "I was delivered an edict: the space allotted to the Psychohormonal Research Unit . . . would be reallocated. The new space would be away from the hospital campus in a commercial building. No further explanation would be given. There would be no appeal. . . . My response was to write this book."

In a 1991 autobiographical essay included in the anthology *The History of Clinical Psychology in Autobiography,* Money continually veered from the subject of his contributions to sexology to revisit his battles with the Johns Hopkins administration. Angrily evoking the termination of his human sexology course, Money wrote, "What the students at Johns Hopkins have lost has become the gain of students around the world. For them I now have more time to write." In the same essay, Money excoriated the (unnamed) Paul McHugh as "the most contentiously destructive person I have ever known" and gloated that "[h]is clandestine efforts to get rid of me failed." Money portrayed his current diminished status in the grim and dangerous basement setting of the Psychohormonal Research Unit with not untypical grandiloquence. "Working as an off-campus exile," he wrote, "in a green subterranean jungle that flourishes under artificial light, I have a sense of kinship with dissidents like Galileo, who by order of the Vatican lived as an exile under house arrest."

Inevitably, perhaps, in the same essay Money addressed those in the field of sexual development who had challenged his scientific theories over the years. Though he did not mention Milton Diamond by name, there was little doubt that the University of Hawaii professor was high on the list of those whom Money now castigated for "shamelessly" attacking him. Yet after lambasting these critics, Money segued into a tone of lofty Olympian remove, finally dismissing his academic disputants as beneath his notice. "My personal impression," he wrote, "is that they are lacking in the special talent for original thinking, for formulating new concepts and hypotheses, and for making new discoveries." Of his continued academic survival, Money wrote, "I have survived by putting into practice my own maxim and have not been lured into declaring a war that I had no possible chance of winning. Instead of mounting a direct counterattack, I would adopt a policy of disengagement and redirect my energies into an alternative channel of achievement."

Money put into effect just such a strategy of disengagement six years later, in the spring of 1997, when his career and reputation suffered their greatest blow to date, from the worldwide media response to Diamond and Sigmundson's paper on the twins case. To the many news organizations that requested comment from him about the now-infamous case, the psychologist refused to speak, citing confidentiality laws. I was among the raft of reporters who sought an interview with Money (for the article I was preparing for *Rolling Stone*). In a letter, I urged him to speak with me, and assured him that I would treat the story with scrupulous objectivity. He declined, but over the ensuing weeks and months, we exchanged a number of e-mails in which he eventually offered to work with me as a kind of silent collaborator on what he called "a piece of investigative journalism." He offered to supply me with the requisite reprints from his published work and to vet my unpublished article to "check the accuracy of some data."

This invitation was withdrawn in late August. Having returned from a second trip to Winnipeg, I notified Money for the first time that I had located and interviewed the patient and his family and had furthermore secured David's promise of a signed confidentiality waiver freeing Money to speak to me about the case. Money's tone changed abruptly. From would-be silent collaborator, he now grew ice-cold. "Thank you for your e-mail of August 24th, to which my reply is that my position has not changed and will not change," he wrote. "I am not under any circumstances available for an interview regarding the Reimer case, and have no further comments to make. So please desist."

I did desist for the next two months while I wrote my *Rolling Stone* story. In early November, with the article going to press, I phoned Money's office to check some facts with his assistant, William Wang. I was surprised when Money got on the line. Although he refused to discuss David Reimer's case directly, he claimed that the media's reporting of it reflected nothing more than a conservative political bias. He was particularly incensed by the *New York Times* front-page story. "It's part of the antifeminist movement," he said. "They say masculinity and femininity are built into the genes so women should get back to the mattress and the kitchen." As to his failure to report the outcome of the case, Money was unapologetic, repeating his claim that he had lost contact with the Reimers when they did not return to Johns Hopkins and that the opportunity to conduct a follow-up had been denied to him. Money sounded affronted when I suggested to him what various of his defenders had hinted to me: that the misreporting of the case was all the Reimers' fault and that David's mother, in particular, in her zeal to believe in the experiment's success—and to please Money—had given him a "rosy picture."

"I was *not* being given a rosy picture," he said irritably, as if stung by the suggestion that he would have failed to factor in any such maternal bias in his assessment of the case's progress. "The only thing that was of importance to me was that I didn't get *any* picture at all after the family simply stopped coming to Johns Hopkins."

He stood by his original reporting of the case and dismissed my suggestion that he "misperceived" what was going on with the child in their one-on-one sessions. Furthermore, he implied that David's reversion to his biological sex might not have been entirely his own decision. "I have no idea," Money said, "how much he was coached in what he wanted, since I haven't seen the person." He also hinted that Diamond and Sigmundson's paper had a hidden agenda. "There is no reason I should have been excluded from the follow-up, was there?" he asked. "Someone had a knife in my back. But it's not uncommon in science. The minute you stick your head up above the grass, there's a gunman ready to shoot you." Told of these comments, Diamond says that he had repeatedly invited Money to share or publish information on the twins over the previous fifteen years, always to no avail.

When I asked Money about Diamond's appeal to delay surgery on intersexual babies until they are old enough to speak for themselves, Money grew angry. Apparently forgetting the conclusions he had reached in his own Harvard thesis review of over two hundred and fifty untreated intersexes, he emphatically rejected the idea that a person could survive a childhood with ambiguous genitalia. "I've seen the people who were the victim of that," he said. "I've heard these poor people describe how they had to sit in a locked room and not go out for fear that someone would see them." Money insisted that surgical intervention at the earliest opportunity after birth was the only guarantee of the child's future happiness. "You cannot be an *it*," he declared, adding that Diamond's recommendations would lead intersexes back to the days when they locked themselves away in shame and worked as "circus freaks."

Money refused to discuss any aspect of his personal life. "You're trying to entrap me," he said, darkly. "Just like my patients try to entrap me."

At this point Money seemed determined to get off the phone. Before he did so, I reminded him that his now classic text, *Man & Woman, Boy & Girl*, was still in print and that it reports the twins case as a success. I asked if it would not be worthwhile for him to make changes in the text for a future edition. Money said flatly, "I'll be dead by then."

Despite its ring of finality, this proved not to be Money's last word on the case. After the publication of my *Rolling Stone* story in December 1997, he again broke his press silence when he granted an interview to a sympathetic writer and friend, Michael King, in the New Zealand magazine *The Listener*. There Money dismissed both Diamond and Sigmundson's John/Joan paper and my *Rolling Stone* article as part of a dark conspiracy against him. The *Listener* article furthermore hinted that David and his family were deliberately lying about Brenda's life for financial gain, since David had decided to collaborate on this book, and moviemakers had expressed interest in the saga. King's article described Money as "surprisingly resilient and sanguine" despite the controversy and ended with news of the undimmed status that

Money still enjoys among U.S. funding agencies. "He has recently been recommended for a grant from the National Institutes of Health for a major new project, a classification and consolidation of contemporary knowledge of paraphilias or 'perversions,'" King reported. I checked with the NIH in the summer of 1999 and learned that Money is still supported by the same NIH research grant that he was awarded in the mid-1950s. His most recent renewal was in the amount of $135,956.

Nor does Money lack for defenders within the academic community—and in particular among professors of psychology, many of whose tenured positions and clinical appointments have been built upon the promulgation and dissemination of Money's theories of psychosexual development. One of his more engaging and intelligent defenders is Dr. Kenneth Zucker, a psychologist at the Clarke Institute of Psychiatry in Toronto and a longtime adherent to Money's nurturist bias in gender identity formation. (In his clinical work, Zucker has for years attempted to modify homosexuality and transexualism in boy and girl children.) Several months after the publication of Diamond and Sigmundson's article, Zucker wrote a paper entitled "Experiment of Nurture," which was framed as a direct response to the John/Joan revelations. Showing his environmentalist leanings, Zucker suggested that the twins case had failed not because David possessed a male biology, but because of certain "psychosocial factors"—in particular "parental ambivalence regarding the initial decision to reassign the infant as a girl."

Efforts on the part of Money's defenders to blame the failure of the case on Ron's and Janet's supposed lack of commitment were by no means exclusive to Zucker; many of Money's acolytes have made the same charge to me in interviews. These charges might carry more weight if not for the fact that all the evidence shows that Ron and Janet were almost slavishly devoted to the experiment—not to mention that Money himself, in his reports on the case, repeatedly described Ron and Janet as particularly skilled and committed parents in the rearing of their daughter. To be sure, once news of the case's failure emerged, rumors apparently originating with Money leaked into the scientific community that Ron and Janet were rural fundamentalists whose restricted religious and cultural values had made it impossible for them to accept their child's sex change in the first place, and that therefore they unconsciously undermined it. In reality, Ron and Janet grew up and spent the majority of their lives in the modern metropolis of Winnipeg (except for the three teen years they spent on farms), and both had (like Money himself) thoroughly rejected the fundamentalist religion of their parents (so much so that they refused even to be married in a Mennonite church). All new claims to the contrary, neither Ron nor Janet labored under outmoded stereotypes of men's and women's roles which would have forbidden them from accepting a merely "tomboyish" daughter, nor was their surrounding community of 1970s Winnipeg—an eclectic, cosmopolitan mix of cultures, religions, backgrounds, races, and socioeconomic levels—predisposed to rejecting a girl who did not conform to rigid stereotypes of femininity.

Zucker's paper, however, did not concern itself solely with unnamed "psychosocial factors" that supposedly negatively influenced the case. He also presented a long-term follow-up on a second case of a developmentally normal baby boy who had been raised as a girl. In a shocking parallel to David's case, this child (also, coincidentally, a Canadian) had lost his penis to a bungled circumcision by electrocautery and had subsequently been castrated and reassigned as a girl at seven months of age in 1971. Now twenty-six years old, the patient was described by Zucker as still living in the female sex. "She denied any uncertainty about being a female from as far back as she could remember," Zucker wrote, "and did not report any dysphoric feelings about being a woman." At the same time, Zucker admitted that the case could not be deemed an unalloyed example of the efficacy of sex reassignment, for he was obliged to acknowledge that the patient, in childhood, had always enjoyed "stereotypically masculine toys and games"; that as an adult she works in a " 'blue collar' job practiced almost exclusively by men"; and that she is currently living with a woman, in her third significant sexual relationship with a member of the female sex.

Nevertheless, Zucker concluded, "In this case . . . the experiment of nurture was successful regarding female gender identity differentiation," and he cited the case as convincing proof that her rearing as a girl "overrode any putative influences of a normal prenatal masculine sexual biology."

Struck by the seeming incongruity of these conclusions, I spoke with Zucker about the case at his office in Toronto in the summer of 1998. Our conversation only served to raise further doubts about the paper's conclusions, for Zucker was unable to answer any of my specific questions about whether the patient might not have been telling the researchers what they wanted to hear when she stated that she had never harbored any doubts about her gender. By now I understood that this is a phenomenon endemic to all areas of sex research that rely on patient testimony, but particularly so in the fraught and sensitive world of sex reassignment, where as one ISNA member told me, "You feel so embarrassed and ashamed to be talking to someone that you'll basically tell them *anything* so you can get the hell out of there." Zucker agreed that such scenarios are not unfamiliar, but he couldn't say whether such a dynamic was at work in the case in question. And for a simple reason. He had never met the patient and had based his reporting solely on information supplied to him by the people listed as coauthors of the paper. These included a gynecologist with no training in the assessment of gender identity, and a psychiatrist who had conducted only two interviews with the woman—the first when she was sixteen, the second when she was twenty-six.

There was, as well, further reason to feel uneasy about the paper's conclusions, and this had to do with its murky provenance. It was only in the closing moments of my interview with Zucker, after I had turned off my tape recorder, that he let fall that the paper had another silent collaborator—an investigator who, when notified of the researchers' efforts, had hastened to supply records he had gathered on the patient in her early childhood. The investigator was John Money, who had authorized and overseen the patient's sex reassignment in infancy and who had, true to practice, conducted a number of annual follow-ups with the child until she (for reasons unspecified in Zucker's paper) stopped returning to Johns Hopkins.

16

≡

IT HAS BEEN TWENTY YEARS since Brenda Reimer made her transformation to David. That metamorphosis marked a turning point in the family's fortunes. Ron, who had been struggling to get his business on its feet, began finally to build a faithful clientele of construction companies and factories. By the early 1980s he was earning forty thousand dollars a year, the best money he had made in his life. Janet continued to see her psychiatrist, and by the mid-1980s, with lithium treatment, her depressions had abated. "I found out what kind of person I really was," she says. "And I went to my children and apologized to them. I said, 'I know at times I was unreasonable and that you were wary of me sometimes because you didn't know what was going to come up next, and you didn't altogether trust me or feel you could take me into your confidence.' I told them that I felt great remorse."

The improvements in Ron's finances and Janet's emotional health brought a harmony the couple hadn't known since the earliest days of their marriage. "I would lay down my life for Ron," Janet told me in the summer of 1998. "Actually, I remember something Dr. Money once said to me. He said, 'I don't know why people always say *making love*; it's *making sex*.' Back then I didn't have an answer for him. Now I do. What I have with Ron is love. We make *love*."

Neither Ron nor Janet pretends that they can ever put the past behind them completely. Janet remains the more talkative on the subject of the guilt and grief that are the main emotions associated with their decision, thirty years ago, to turn their son into a daughter. Ron typically finds it more difficult to speak directly about these matters, but he communicates them nevertheless in his more spare and diffident speech.

"I wonder," I asked him in our first interview, "if you've ever got to a point where you forgot this had happened?"

Ron shook his head. "No," he said. "We never forget." Then he said it again. "Never forget." And once more: "Never forget."

I remembered a notation I had seen in Dr. Ingimundson's psychiatric notes from the spring of 1977 concerning a private meeting with Janet and Ron. Under the heading "Counter transference" (the psychoanalytic term for the emotions experienced by the therapist toward the patient), Ingimundson had written, "Have a need to protect them." I now felt something of the same need.

"I know David doesn't blame you at all," I told Ron. "He attributes all the best things in his life to you and Janet."

Ron smiled weakly and blinked away the moisture in his eyes. "I'm glad *he* feels that way," Ron said. "I don't know if *I* feel like that."

Perhaps the greatest insight that Ron gave me into his emotions concerning the failed experiment came when our formal interview was over, and we repaired from the backyard to the house. Ron poured us a pair of Crown Royal rye whiskeys, then invited me to watch a tape of his favorite movie. It had been a long day, and I told him I would probably head back to my Travelodge and turn in early. Ron was strangely, and uncharacteristically, insistent. "This is a really great movie," he said. "I got Brian to tape it for me off HBO. I've seen it maybe twenty times." The movie, he said, was called *Crossroads*. I soon realized that it was pointless to resist; by now Janet (who also loved the movie) had joined Ron in his entreaties. So I followed them to the basement, where we settled down in front of the television set.

I vaguely registered the movie's plot as it played on the Reimers' TV screen. Ralph Macchio plays a cocky young blues guitarist who befriends an eighty-year-old blues player, one Blind Willie Brown. Together the pair travel from New York City to Blind Willie's Mississippi home, where he has some "unfinished business" to take care of. As Ry Cooder's keening blues guitar soundtrack wailed over the opening credits, Janet turned to me and said, "We love this music. I think you have to have been to hell and back to love the blues." In its detail, and in the thorny, affectionate relationship between the older and the younger man, the movie was better than I expected; but I still found myself fighting off sleep as the saga reached its final act, which occurs at a stark, dusty crossroads in the depths of rural Mississippi—at which point I began to grow alert.

Drawing on the famous legend of blues guitarist Robert Johnson (who was said to have won his skills as a guitar player from a deal he signed with the devil at "the crossroads"), the movie now revealed that Blind Willie Brown had made a similar deal almost sixty years earlier, when he was seventeen years old. But Blind Willie had not become famous and celebrated. Instead he had ended up destitute in a Harlem old folks' home. Now he had come for a reckoning. Standing in the shadow of a leafless tree at the crossroads, he watched as the dapper, smooth-talking, grinning man with whom he had struck his deal all those years ago materialized from nowhere. The two men face each other. Ron, who was sitting in an armchair to my right, set down his rye and 7-Up and sat forward a little, bringing his face closer to the screen.

Confronting the man who had hoodwinked him into his bum deal, Willie Brown demands that the Man in Black tear up the contract between them—"and give me some peace."

The Man in Black laughs derisively. "Why on earth would I want to do that?" he asks.

Willie is outraged at the man's insouciance. "*You* sloughed up on *your* end of things," Willie shouts. "I didn't end up where I wanted. I didn't end up with *nothing*—didn't get nothing!"

But the grinning Man in Black offers no apologies. "Ain't nothing *ever* as good as we want it to be!"

Both Ron and Janet hung on every word of this dialogue— as if they expected that on this viewing, the scene might finally play out differently. When the scene ended, Ron sat back in his chair, then glanced quickly at me and away. Several times during our long interview that day, I had tried to get Ron to speak about how he now felt about John Money and the momentous decision he had convinced Ron and Janet to make. He had made a few halting, stumbling efforts to answer my question but had clearly failed to say all that was in him. Now I felt I had my answer. Along with Ron's grief and guilt there was an obvious admixture of outraged betrayal, which lay too deep for him to express in words.

Nor were those emotions solely confined to the way Ron and Janet felt about the son they had agreed to convert into a daughter. For David was by no means the only casualty of that doomed experiment. The matched control, too, had suffered, and suffered badly, with results that were still being felt. Brian's episode of shoplifting in the spring before the family's flight to British Columbia proved not to be an isolated incident, but a precursor of more serious transgressions to come.

"I was thirteen when I got involved with a bad crowd," Brian explains. "It started with drinking and smoking, and it eventually wound up into stealing cars and dope and fighting. For me, personally, I never got into armed robbery and I never really hurt anyone that bad. . . ." Then Brian thinks for a moment and amends that. "One person I hurt pretty bad." He is referring to a boy whose arm he broke so severely in a fight that he was called to court. Listening to the litany of Brian's brutal and criminal acts as a teen and young adult, I was mystified. Even in adulthood he clearly demonstrated, in comparison with David's more conventionally male attitudes, a greater aesthetic awareness and a sensitive side out of keeping with the endless tales of mayhem and brutality that filled his teens and twenties. "That's the side I couldn't show to people," he says. "The sensitive guy finished last. The tough guy gets the respect, and he gets left alone. That's bad to say, but that's the reality of it. He gets all the girlfriends; he gets invited to all the parties."

Being included by his friends was vitally important for Brian because of the abandonment he felt from his parents. "I had problems growing up, but they had to deal with my sister's problems, which were so much bigger," Brian says. "But try growing up all your life feeling that your problems are nothing."

Brian learned about his sister's true birth status from Janet on 14 March 1980—the same day that Ron told Brenda.

"My mother was working at the parking lot," Brian says. "She called me and said, 'Brian, I have to talk to you about something.' So I visited her at work, in this booth where she sat. We were having coffee. She said, 'It's about Brenda.' Then she says, 'Brenda was really your brother.' And I got upset."

Brian's reaction was typically explosive. He jumped from his chair and smashed his fist into the booth's reinforced glass window. "I broke both panes," Brian recalls. "I was pissed off. Then I cooled down, and mother told me everything that had happened—about the circumcision and everything. I said, 'Now I can understand. I can put the pieces of the puzzle together. It makes sense now.' But I felt, 'Shit, the first fourteen years of my life was a *lie*.'"

And there would be other emotional hurdles for Brian to get over—which became clear later that same day, when he saw his twin for the first time since hearing the news. "Dave was wearing a suit," Brian recalls. "He says, 'What d'you think?' I said, 'Hey. You look good. I'm happy for you.'" But Brian admits that David's transformation brought mixed emotions. In the past, Brian had always had his status as the family's only son to make him feel special. Now even that was gone. "I supported him one hundred percent," Brian says. "I felt a sense of relief because now he finally fitted into society. At the same time, I'm not big brother anymore."

Just how deeply affected Brian was by this swift and emotionally bewildering turn of events was clear a year later, shortly before the twins' sixteenth birthday and two weeks before David underwent his first phalloplasty, when on 17 June 1981, Brian was taken to the emergency room of St. Boniface Hospital to have his stomach pumped. He had drunk from a bottle of drain cleaner. At the time, Brian told his family that the suicide gesture was over a girl who had broken up with him. Today Brian admits that was not the truth. "Mom was worried sick about David," he says. "Every waking moment was David. It was 'Brian's OK, he can take care of himself.' Any problem I had seemed trivial compared to David's. So it was almost like I had to do *something* to get a little bit of attention."

At sixteen, to his parents' consternation, Brian quit school and took a job pumping gas. He moved out of the house and started living with a girlfriend. At nineteen, Brian married her, and had two children. The marriage proved tumultuous and ended in acrimony and divorce a few years later.

Brian's life reached its nadir after the divorce. Unemployed and trying to raise his children as a single father, he began to drink to excess and suffered bouts of severe depression. His children were temporarily removed from his custody and lived for six months with Ron and Janet. During that time Brian cleaned himself up and got control of his life. In the early 1990s he landed a well-paid union job working a lathe in a metal-spinning factory. He remarried, had a daughter, and moved into a house he bought in Winnipeg's West End. Prozac has helped with his mood swings.

Aside from his wife and children, Brian says that the person he knows best in the world is his brother. Despite the lingering rivalries that sometimes drive the twins, even in adulthood, to severe periods of feuding and dissension, they remain extraordinarily attuned to one another's inner lives. Yet Brian admits that, like his parents, he harbors guilt about David. It is a guilt that dates back roughly to sixth grade at Agassiz Drive school, when Brian pulled away from his social pariah sister. "I had a choice," Brian says. "I could be with my friends or with my sister. They made it quite clear—subtle but clear—that I had a choice." He chose to have friends—a choice for which he has never fully forgiven himself. "I wanted to have a life," he says. "I turned my back on Brenda." Only many years later, after David had been living in his true sex for almost five years, would the brothers again grow close.

At our first meeting, in late June 1997, Brian proudly cataloged the striking similarities between them, likening David and himself to those cases of identical twins separated at birth and who, when reunited in adulthood, discover that their lives bear uncanny parallels. "Both me and Dave married in September," he told me. "Both have one dog and one cat. Both are factory workers. Both make around the same amount of money. We both like to watch *Biography*, 20/20, *Fifth Estate*, 60 *Minutes*. Both love Elvis. In a way, it's always been me and my brother against the world."

More than two decades have passed since David Reimer had his final contact with Dr. John Money, when the famous sexologist slipped him fifteen dollars in his parents' living room. In the intervening years, David often fantasized about what he might say or do to the psychologist if they were ever to meet face-to-face. He admits that as a younger man his fantasies ran to violence. No more. Determined to get on with his life, he refuses to dwell on a past that he cannot change. In their paper, Diamond and Sigmundson describe David as a "forward-looking person." In conversation, Diamond calls him a true hero. And indeed, David's life today defies the dire prognosis of the psychiatrist who thirty-three years ago declared that he would never marry and "must live apart." At the same time, it has been impossible for him to put the past away entirely. Over the course of our interviews together, David spoke with a blunt and unvarnished honesty about his extraordinary childhood and youth. He spoke without self-pity. His sufferings were extreme, his survival almost miraculous: both lend to his unschooled speech an aura of oracular wisdom.

"I don't blame my parents," he told me. "A lot of people are going to be surprised by that. They'd have to put themselves in my situation and live out my life, knowing that my parents have sacrificed so much. My dad's a very special man. He's got a lot in his heart, and he doesn't know how to express himself. But you know, you can see in the soul of his eyes that he's hurting and that he cares and he loves you.

"My mother is a lot better, she's getting help. She admits that she did wrong things. Some people wouldn't even do that. You know, as a very little kid I had a crush on my mother. I used to pick dandelions for her. She was the most beautiful woman in the whole world to me.

"When I think of my brother as a kid, I see this little seven-year-old with a bean shave, puppy-dog eyes, asking for help. 'Help me! Help me!' He'd get into trouble, get into a fight, and I'd do my best to bail him out. He'd let the scrawniest guy beat the hell out of him. My brother hiding behind me! I'd look ridiculous fighting because of the way I was dressed—I didn't look the part to bail him out. My dad gave me shit when I fought because he thought it put Brian in a position where *he* would have to try to protect *me*. 'It's unfair to put your brother in a position like that.' I tried to explain: 'This is not my *brother's* fight, this is *my* fight.' It didn't do any good. I'm not going to take anything away from Brian: he had it rough because of me. But it was directed at *me*, not him. When they picked on him, they were making fun of me. 'There's your butch sister.'

"My childhood. It comes to me. I don't go and think about it. I'm trying to sleep, and these stupid thoughts come into my head, and I shake my head and I say, 'I'm going to think about something else,' but it will jump right back into my head. Memories of how I used to look. Memories of being belittled by my classmates. Memories of just trying to survive.

"If I had grown up as a boy without a penis? Oh, I would still have had my problems, but they wouldn't have been compounded the way they are now. If I was raised a boy, I would have been more accepted by other people. I would have been way better off if they had just left me alone, because when I switched back over, then I had *two* problems on my hands, not just one, because of them trying to brainwash me into accepting myself as a girl. So you got the *psychological* thing going in your head. When I'm intimate with my wife it sometimes *haunts* me. From time to time it gets to flashbacks of you as a kid, and it makes you— I admit, sometimes I have to get up out of the bed and go to the bathroom and throw up.

"You know, if I had lost my arms and my legs and wound up in a wheelchair where you're moving everything with a little rod in your mouth—would that make me less of a person? It just seems that they implied that you're nothing if your penis is gone. The second you lose *that,* you're nothing, and they've got to do surgery and hormones to turn you into something. Like you're a zero. It's like your whole personality, everything about you is all directed—all pinpointed— toward what's between the legs. And to me, that's ignorant. I don't have the kind of education that these scientists and doctors and psychologists have, but to me it's very ignorant. If a woman lost her breasts, do you turn her into a guy? To make her feel 'whole and complete'?

"I feel sorry for women. I've been there. 'You're a little lady—go into the kitchen.' Or 'We don't want you to chop wood—you might hurt yourself.' I remember when I was a kid and women were fighting like hell to get equal rights. I said, 'Good for them.' I kind of sensed what position women had in society. Way down there. And that's how I was portrayed. And I didn't want to go way down there. I felt, I can do what anybody else can! But 'Oh, you're a girl—you might get hurt playing ball.'

"At Agassiz Drive school there was this guy, Tubby Wayne.

He was a male chauvinist pig. 'Women are dirt; they can't do anything men can do.' He kept saying, 'You don't know anything. You're a *girl*; girls don't know anything.' So I finally said to him, 'You think you're so tough? Then hit me. C'mon hit me.' He says, 'No, I'm not going to hit you; you're a girl.' 'No. Hit me. I'm not going to put up with this.' He wouldn't, so I punched him—and he laughed at me. It was a good thing he didn't hit me, I guess. But I was thinking, Don't hide behind the 'I don't hit girls' excuse.

"The guys at work don't know about what happened to me. I mean, I work in a *slaughterhouse*. All men. Can you imagine?—'There's the freak who wore dresses as a kid.' They give you that male chauvinist crap all the time. Like they're always saying that they're the *boss* at home. They look at me and ask me, 'Who's the boss?' I say, 'Look, man, in my home it's a partnership. It doesn't mean I wimp out; sometimes I get my way, and sometimes I don't get my way. But either way, it's a partnership.' I mean, who wants a woman with no brains, who follows you blindly? That's more like a slave than a wife. You don't want a slave, you want somebody with her own opinions, somebody who puts you on the right track, someone to show you the right direction. It's very hard to talk to somebody who's stone-cold stupid, who follows you blindly.

"But you know, if I had had a normal life, and none of this had ever happened to me, I'd probably be one of these chauvinistic kind of guys, where the guy goes to work, breaks his back, comes home, and sucks down a beer and watches sports. And if I saw someone like *me* out on TV, I'd sit there saying, 'Oh God that's sick.' That's how I would be. So knowing that that person is *me,* you can realize how sick *I* feel looking back on all this. You wish to God you could switch places with anybody.

"After I tried to kill myself, they put me in one of those psy-

cho wards. Right away they want to put you in a group meeting. You can't even face this by *yourself,* and they're going to
stick you in a room full of people so you can discuss this with
strangers? There was this doctor there who kept telling me that
it was wrong for me to try to kill myself. Well, it's easy for him
to sit there and say, 'Shame, shame, shame.' This guy's been
putting himself through college, he's got a degree, probably living in a fancy house, he's got 2.2 kids, got a normal life. Don't
compare that to me. Not the same.

"I'm happiest when I'm alone. Doesn't mean I'm not
friendly. It's just I'm more comfortable when I'm by myself.
It's not lonely. It's relaxing. It's soothing. It reminds me of my
grandfather's farm. If I go for a walk there, I'm in total peace.
I'm never alone there. You always feel like you're surrounded
in a place like that. Surrounded by what, I don't know. But
you're not alone.

"I still wonder from time to time what it would have been
like to have a biological child: to see how much of me that child
would have. It's not really an ego trip. It's just . . . you feel that
way. But I love my kids, and they're my children—not just my
*step*children. I'm going to want to tell my kids about what happened. I couldn't keep something like this away from them. I'd
feel very uncomfortable about that. I already told my eldest,
when she was fifteen. She had that look on her face, like, 'You
wore *dresses?*' But all in all, she took it well. She said, 'I don't
love you any less, Dad.' I know my middle child would understand, but I won't tell her for years. I have to wait until she's a
lot older. My son? I'll tell him when he's about fifteen.

"I live my life through my son. Everything my son does,
that's *me.* When my son has a little crush on a girl, and he's
leaning on a fence, and the girl comes up and says, 'Hi,' and he's
got that blush thing happening; when he's in Cub Scouts—
that's *me.* I live through him. When he succeeds, that's like *me*

succeeding. Some psychiatrist would disagree with me living my life through him, but I never had any kind of a childhood.

"It's going to be harder to tell my son than to tell my girls. You never know with boys and their fathers. He might think differently about me. You know: 'My father wore dresses, my father had a girl's name, my father lived as a girl.' I mean that's a lot to swallow. You can tell when it's hard for somebody to accept something or is embarrassed. And for him to look at me sideways . . .

"I'm sick to death of feeling ashamed of myself. That feeling will never go away. I did nothing wrong, but it's like you're conditioned to feel ashamed of yourself. The very thought that I was wearing a dress, having a girl's name—the long hair and everything—I'm going to have to carry that for the rest of my life. You can't erase memories like that. I just survive as best I can. Keep telling myself, 'It's not my fault. Not my fault what happened.'

"Mom and Dad wanted this to work so I'd be happy. That's every parent's dream for their child. But I couldn't be happy for my parents. I had to be happy for me. You can't be something that you're not. You have to be *you*."

Embarking on my interviews with David, I had been warned by his former psychiatrist Doreen Moggey that I was engaging in a dangerous psychological process. She feared that David could not negotiate the leap from his current life to his former one without risk of serious mental upset, and urged me to tread gingerly when guiding him back to the memories and events he had tried, for so long, to forget. I heeded her advice, but in my conversations with David—which often stretched to six hours at a sitting, going deep into the small hours of the morning—I found that he bridled at the cautious circumspection of my questioning. He seemed to want nothing more than to charge fearlessly into the past, to speak without restraint about all that had happened to him, to put his true life story on the permanent record, and thus to reclaim it as his own. I also discovered that he wished to reclaim his life not only in the abstract form of interviews with me.

In mid-January 1998 I located and spoke to his old friend Heather Legarry. She still lived in Winnipeg but was married now with a different last name, and she worked as a kindergarten teacher. As was the case in all the interviews I did with those who had known Brenda as a child (and to whom David had authorized me to tell his medical history), I did not at first tell her the truth of Brenda's birth, so as not to color her memories and impressions of the girl; but when I did finally reveal to her that Brenda had been born a boy and now lived as a man named David, she said that she would like to see him. Recalling how David had once dodged a confrontation with Heather at the Go-Cart track fifteen years earlier, I wondered how he would greet this news. I was surprised when David said that he would like to see her, too. That Sunday they met privately and had lunch, while I stayed home with Jane and helped her nurse her mostly-mock jealousy—a jealousy that became a little more real when David failed to return home for almost four hours. When he did arrive, he (with typical thoughtfulness) bore a red rose for his wife, but he also bore an expression, on his face, that I had never seen before; it was a look of serene and somehow euphoric peacefulness. Asked by Jane what they had talked about for *so long*, David even got off a joke about his horrendous past. "Oh," he said, "just *girl talk!*" In fact, he later said, he and Heather had discussed all aspects of his childhood, comparing notes on their shared memories, reexamining their old friendship in the light of what neither had known at the time. It was a meeting that had clearly removed from David a burden that had weighed on him for almost two decades.

None of which is to say that revisiting David's past with him for the purposes of researching this book was not without its painful, and precarious, moments—particularly when I stumbled upon one last family secret of the Reimers' that had never been exposed: one of the white lies that Janet had constantly been obliged to concoct for Brenda in order to quell her daughter's suspicions about her true identity; a white lie that had, through parental oversight, never been corrected with David, and which thus lay buried for almost twenty years, like an unexploded land mine.

On my first ever trip to Winnipeg, eight months earlier, one of the first things David had ever told me about his mother was that she was a published poet. He described to me, with touching pride, how he had actually met the editors of the journal that had printed his mother's work. I soon learned, of course, that the story of Janet as poet was a ruse. Wanting to learn from David his impressions of meeting the BBC reporters on that day in October 1979, I did not feel comfortable keeping up the fiction that they were poetry editors. I knew that I would have to explode the lie. I put it off for as long as I could, until close to the end of my monthlong stay in Winnipeg in early 1998. I tried to break the news gently, but David still reacted very badly to this jarring revelation.

"Why did I have to find out *this* way?" he raged. "I'm a thirty-two-year-old man!"

For the next two hours he railed against his mother's "gutlessness" in not telling him the truth; he shouted that he had been lied to all his life, and said, "You don't expect that from the people you trust and love!" His anger and upset were frighteningly intense, but thankfully David's fury soon burnt itself down, and the next day he visited his mother and spoke to her about the deception. She apologized for having overlooked this final lie, and they made up over it. In the end, the exposure of that last, lingering falsehood had a positive effect, Janet said, in removing an obstacle that had persisted from David's childhood of secrets and lies. I was glad, and relieved, of this outcome, but at the same time, glimpsing David's apocalyptic rage made me wish, not for the first time, that he could bring himself to see a therapist, if only to vent the combustible anger that periodically built up in him over his past.

But David's dismal experience with the mental health profession as a child has guaranteed that he will never consult a psychiatrist in adulthood—unless it were his old friend, Mary McKenty, and that is impossible, given that she, at age eighty-three, has long since retired. Still, David and she have remained friends, and he accompanied me on a visit I made to her home in June 1998, on my final trip to Winnipeg. Though now in the grip of Alzheimer's disease, and often unable even to recognize her own children, McKenty knew David immediately. She was a tiny woman with long, gray hair and the masklike expression typical of Alzheimer's sufferers, but her face blossomed into a delighted smile when she saw David step over the threshold of her door.

While David chatted with Mary's live-in nurses, I retired with her to a small sitting room off the front hall. Fortunately, we had come on a day when Mary's memory was particularly good, and her answers to my questions, though abbreviated, were spoken in a strong clear voice that left no doubt that she knew precisely what we were talking about.

I asked Mary how she had handled Brenda's difficult case. She shrugged. "I tried to be sensitive and supportive," she said. I asked if Brenda had ever seemed at all like a girl. "No," she said, "not like a girl at all." I recalled to myself Money's claim that Brenda must have been "coached" in rejecting girlhood;

no evidence for this existed anywhere in the local treatment team's notes, and David had been unequivocal in stating that McKenty had in no way "coached" him. But I felt it was my obligation to ask. Had Mary always kept Brenda's true birth status from her? "Yes," she said. I asked if she had tried to steer her gently away from being a girl. "No," McKenty said. "The things were for *her* to realize and for *her* to do."

Impressed with what I had been able to glean about Mary's special human touch with her patients—and especially with Brenda—I asked her about her general approach to psychiatry. In reply, she said "You have a parental attitude to your patients." Then she glanced in the direction of the hallway, where David's voice could be heard. "Just like a parent," she added, "you often admire them." I was moved by this word *admire*—so different from what one ordinarily expects to hear a psychiatrist say about a patient, or to hear a highly educated doctor like McKenty say about a slaughterhouse sanitation worker like David Reimer. But it was clear that her admiration for David was total.

I asked if she had ever read any of John Money's work. Her face, which had been eerily immobile, crumpled into a scowl. "Yes," she said with clear distaste. I asked what she thought of it. "I thought it was *unusual*," she said dryly.

David came into the room. She immediately brightened. He crouched down on the carpet in front of where she sat on the sofa.

"It's been a long time, Mary," he said gently.

"How long has it been?"

"Ten years at least."

"And it's been almost twenty since Mary started treating you," I said.

David looked sheepish. Just that morning, he and I had been looking at Mary's therapy notes with Brenda, and

David had been aghast to be reminded of the cruel tricks he had played on her in their earliest sessions. He apologized to her now. "I drew a nasty picture of you," he said. "I took you hostage with a toy gun."

"I didn't mind," she said.

"I made a Death Warrant in your name!"

Mary laughed and pretended to reach for her cane. "You'd better watch it!" she said. Then Mary grew serious and looked at David. His smile faded, too. For a moment it might have been twenty years ago, and the two might have been patient and doctor again. And indeed, Mary's next utterance was a classic psychiatric inquiry, a question that went to the very heart of the psychotherapeutic enterprise, and to the heart, for that matter, of the universal enterprise of becoming a self-realized human being—the enterprise upon which we are all engaged.

"Is there anything you want to change?" she asked.

David looked down at his hands. He breathed a tired sigh. Then he looked at her. He smiled. "Everything I've wanted to do," he said, "I've done."

Among the things that David Reimer has done that give him greatest pride is his decision to speak out publicly about his ordeal, and the positive changes that have resulted from that act.

For despite the brave efforts of Cheryl Chase, despite the three decades that Milton Diamond spent trying to warn doctors about the dangers in current management of intersex conditions, despite the long-term follow-up of sex-reassigned youngsters in Bill Reiner's study, the medical establishment remained reluctant to address the issue. But in October 1998, amid the growing controversy ignited by Diamond and Sigmundson's "John/Joan" article, the American Academy of Pediatrics invited Diamond to address its prestigious annual meeting of urologists. Diamond spoke about the failed twins case and spelled out his and Sigmundson's revised protocols for the treatment of children with irregular or injured genitals. His speech was met with sustained applause from the physicians—the first tangible sign that the medical establishment as a whole might be prepared to alter what, for the past four decades, has been the accepted standard of care. It was a moment of triumph that Diamond declines to accept for himself, and instead directly attributes to the willingness of David Reimer to speak out about his extraordinary life as one of medicine's most famous, if unwitting, guinea pigs.

In speaking out, David has shaken to its foundations the clinical practice founded on John Money's work; he has also raised profound questions about a theory that has held sway for most of the twentieth century: Freud's theory that a child's healthy psychological development as boy or a girl rests on the presence or absence of the penis—the ultimate reason that David was converted to girlhood in the first place. It is a notion that today is also being called into question by neurobiological research, which is leading scientists toward the conclusion that, as Dr. Reiner says, "the most important sex organ is not the genitals; it's the brain."

David Reimer puts it another way when he speaks of his pride in his role as husband, father, and sole breadwinner in the family he never believed he would be lucky enough to have. "From what I've been taught by my father," he says, "what makes you a man is you treat your wife well, you put a roof over your family's head, you're a good father. Things like that add up much more to being a man than just *bang-bang-bang*—sex. I guess John Money would consider my children's biological fathers to be real men. But they didn't stick around to take care of the children. I did. That, to me, is a man."

Epilogue

≡

IT IS ONE OF THE FIRST MAXIMS of science that no theory can be based on a single experiment. This truism applies as much to Milton Diamond's revelations about the failure of the twins case as it does (or *should* have) to Money's original reporting of its success. While it is also true that Diamond cites David's case *not* as an isolated one (he has repeatedly presented evidence to the same effect, both clinical and theoretical, in cases involving intersexes), it is only through continued study and follow-up on cases of developmentally normal boys turned into girls that medical science can confidently proclaim whether it is nature or nurture that predominates in the making of men and women, boys and girls.

Such cases, which rely exclusively on genital accidents resulting in loss of the penis, are necessarily rare. Yet with the high-profile debate generated by David's case, there are already signs that what cases *do* exist are being followed up and reported on with a greater rigor than previously. In February

1998 the *Urology Times* published a report by Dr. Bernardo Ochoa, former chief of pediatric and urologic surgery at the University of Antioquia in Medellín, Colombia, on the case of a baby boy who, like David, lost his penis in an injury and was subsequently reassigned to girlhood by castration, vaginal surgery, and hormone treatment—with results strikingly similar to David's. "She and her family received extensive psychosocial assistance," Ochoa reported. "However, when she became an adolescent, 14 years later, she demanded to be reassigned as a boy because she didn't feel she was a girl."

In pursuit of further data, doctors and researchers will almost certainly pay particularly close attention to events that began at Atlanta's Northside Hospital in 1985, when on a single day two developmentally normal newborn boys suffered severe penile burns from bungled electrocautery circumcisions. One boy lost his penis entirely, the other a significant portion. The parents of the child in the former case agreed to sex reassignment of their child as a female; the other parents opted to have their child receive plastic surgery to create an artificial penis.

Here was another of those one-in-a-million chances, another unplanned experiment of fate, in which two children became ideal matched controls in a living laboratory experiment, this one offering researchers a unique comparison study of how best to deal with the calamity of penile loss: sex reassignment or phalloplasty? With the children currently on the eve of their fourteenth birthdays, privacy issues have prevented much information on their condition from being released, and I was able to glean only minimal reports when I spoke with the several lawyers who represented the parents in their lawsuits against Northside Hospital.

Thomas Sampson is the lawyer who won a $22.8 million settlement for the parents of Antonio, the boy who is being raised as a male. According to Sampson, Antonio is doing better today than was ever expected at the time of his injury. He experienced a period of difficulty in his early school years, when he underwent several operations for phalloplasty and experienced some cruelty, both intentional and otherwise, from his peers. But now in tenth grade, his social situation is considerably better. He displays no difficulties with his identity as a male, though whether he will ever feel confident enough to have sexual intercourse with his artificial penis and to father his own children, only time will tell.

The fate of the other child is less well known and more carefully guarded. Castrated and converted to girlhood at less than two weeks of age, she is known in court documents simply as "Baby Doe." For the last year and a half, I have sought word of her mental and emotional state from her lawyers and physicians, but they have refused all comment. What few facts I was able to verify independently did not augur particularly well. Her parents divorced while she was still young. Doe lives with her mother—although in a relationship whose future is unsure. According to a lawyer involved in her case, she was recently placed under the care of a court-appointed guardian.

I spoke to David about Baby Doe during my last trip to see him in Winnipeg in the summer of 1998. Deeply upset, he insisted on dictating a letter to the child's parents, in which he offered himself for advice or support to them or their daughter. His letter went unanswered. "I wasn't surprised," David says. "I've been there, and so have my parents. They just need time."

Since then David has found himself dreaming of Doe, who has appeared to him in his sleep as a mute younger sister desperately trying to communicate something through enigmatic scribblings on a child's chalkboard. That David should feel a special kinship with Doe is not surprising, for not only has she undergone the same accident and treatment that have shaped

David's life, she also shares other uncanny similarities with him. Remarkably enough, *both* children injured at Atlanta's Northside Hospital in 1985 happen to have been born on 22 August—twenty years to the day after David and Brian Reimer came into the world. The psychologist who consulted on Baby Doe's case—five years after David announced his decision to live as a male—was Dr. John Money.

Afterword

≡

As its title would suggest, *As Nature Made Him*
places considerable emphasis on the role that biology plays in
the shaping of human sexuality. In that respect, the book was
meant as a clear corrective to the extreme nurturist stance of
the 1960s and 1970s, when biological influences on gender
identity and sexual orientation were dismissed altogether—a
view which still informs much of the thinking of the lay public
even today. For me, learning about the role of prenatal hormones in hardwiring sexual behavior was eye-opening, and a
degree of the urgency I felt in writing the book derived from
the satisfying sense that I was bringing to readers facts probably unknown to them.

Yet while I consider David's case to be among the strongest
evidence yet available for the biological underpinnings of gender, I reject any reading of the book that reduces his story to
simpleminded biological determinism—whether that reduc-
tionism is meant as a compliment to the book, or as a criti-

cism. One reviewer, for instance, praised *As Nature Made Him* for showing that "gender is indeed biologically based and not learned at all." Yet another criticized the book for the same supposed message: "[W]hen it comes to nature-nurture, I believe it's not so much a matter of being right, but a matter of emphasis. A deliberate emphasis on nurture is politically healthier, especially for women." The first statement is preposterous (how can learning play no role "at all" in how an individual comes to understand his position in society?); the second equally so. Political health, or correctness, should play no role in scientific debate—unless, of course, the debate is purely academic theorizing, a kind of intellectual Ping-Pong, in which case nothing rides on it. Unfortunately, within the context of infant sex reassignment, *everything* rides on it, since it is only by continuing to assert nurture's primacy over nature that physicians can continue to assign sexual identities to newborns through surgery, psychological engineering, and hormones. As David's story shows, that is a risky practice indeed.

Happily, the medical profession has, in the wake of the book's publication, shown a heretofore unprecedented willingness to re-examine the practice of infant sex reassignment—and to listen to the testimony of former patients. ISNA founder Cheryl Chase has been invited to speak to the American Academy of Pediatrics, and has joined a group of urologists to form the North American Task Force for Intersexuality, which is collecting long-term data from some two hundred cases of sex-reassigned people and evaluating the long-term effects of the procedure. In May 2000, she spoke at a conference at Johns Hopkins, where she delivered the final talk at the annual meeting of the Lawson Wilkins Pediatric Endocrine Society—perhaps the strongest evidence to date that the medical profession as a whole is willing to reassess the efficacy of infant sex reassignment—and the relative roles of genetics and environment in the making of boys and girls, men and women.

None of this is to suggest that nurture plays no role in gender identity. Virtually every page of *As Nature Made Him* contains an environmental cue or clue that helped to reinforce what Brenda's prenatally virilized brain and nervous system were telling her. Among these environmental cues, I would include the presence of an identical twin brother who so closely resembled Brenda and yet was, mystifyingly, of the opposite sex; the scarred and unfinished state of her genitals which contributed to her conviction that *something* was unusual about her assigned gender; the teasing and ostracization of peers and classmates who jeered at her for her masculinity; the growing realization on the part of Ron and Janet, around the time of Brenda's seventh birthday, that the experiment was a failure; the trips to Johns Hopkins, where her genitals and sexual identity were of such obsessive interest to Money and his students; and indeed, the second-class status assigned to females in society—a condition that leads many dispirited girls to wish (around the time of puberty) that they could be boys. All of these factors, I'm convinced, played a role in undermining the experiment. I attribute the case's final and complete collapse, however, to the pressing insistence of Brenda's biological maleness—her awakening sexual attraction to girls; her inchoate but adamant aversion to possessing breasts and a vagina. For how many children, at the exquisitely awkward age of fourteen, will insist, upon threat of suicide, that they undergo full sex change, in plain view of neighbors, family, and friends? This almost incomprehensible act of courage on Brenda's part speaks more convincingly than any other piece of evidence to the emphatic demands of our biology, and to the necessity that we—all of us—be allowed to live as we feel we must.

Indeed, it was this very courage of David's which was my prime motivation in writing the book. Despite its medical-scientific context, I've always believed that this story transcends the incessant quibbling over the nature/nurture debate. David's is a story about identity in its largest sense—not simply *sexual* identity. His story, for all its uniqueness, is a universal one, and reminds us how it is every person's individual responsibility to define for himself who he is, and to assert that against a world that often opposes, ridicules, oppresses, or undermines him. It is perhaps as much to David's innate will and strength, as it is to his prenatally organized brain and nervous system, that he owes his survival; not many children, at seven years old, could have faced down a man of John Money's famously persuasive temperament. Yet he did so, as he staunchly refused to undergo a surgical procedure (vaginoplasty) which he instinctively knew would seal him into an identity not his own. For me, the emotional crescendo of the story comes in that moment directly after Ron Reimer revealed the stunning truth of her birth to Brenda—and her first question was not about *how* or *why* her parents could have made such a decision; it was not to ask how such a devastating circumcision accident could have occurred. Instead, she asked her birth name. She asked, in effect, *Who am I?* Kept so long from this ultimate knowledge, it was only through learning this essential truth that David was then able to begin assembling a life for himself.

No writer working in the wake of Janet Malcolm's book *The Journalist and the Murderer* can pretend to obliviousness of the many sticky ethical issues surrounding the exploitation of another person's life for the purposes of making one's own living. David Reimer's ordeal, in particular, seemed to highlight these inherent dilemmas of reporting. Not only had he endured sufferings of a singularly private, and potentially embarrassing, nature, but he was also wholly unsophisticated in the ways of publishing. Flying into Winnipeg for the first time in June 1997, I couldn't help but think of Malcolm's "morally indefensible" journalist who swoops into town, coaxes his subjects to reveal their secrets, then departs with his treasure hoard of painful and private facts, which he publishes for his own financial gain and professional advancement.

Hoping to mitigate these unhealthy conditions of journalism, I made two resolutions. First, I promised myself that I would attempt to recount David's experiences in a tone, and within a context, that did not sensationalize them. Second, I arranged to share with David, fifty-fifty, the profits from the book. While this financial arrangement seemed the only proper way to proceed, it introduced the other great ethical dilemma of journalism: the paying of a source. Critics of the practice (and I've always been one of them) point out that sources who agree to speak for money will shape their testimony to fit the perceived needs of the person paying the money. While this is a danger in cases where supermarket tabloids use cash to induce an "insider" to spill dirt on celebrities, I felt we had a quite different situation here. Long before any financial remuneration entered the picture, David had told his story, at length, to Diamond and Sigmundson, who documented it in videotaped interviews; and he had spoken to me, over the course of six months, for my *Rolling Stone* article, without payment of any kind. Given the degree to which his life had already been documented, it would have been easy for me to detect if David were now straying from his story for reasons related to money; furthermore (and perhaps most important), there existed an extensive contemporaneous written record assembled by the various physicians who had treated Brenda since the age of twenty-two months—a record against which all of David's (and his family's) memories could be checked; my extra interviews with a raft of teachers, old classmates, and others close to the family further guaranteed that the Reimers' account of their ordeal was as accurate as possible and untainted by the monetary reward that had now entered the picture. But perhaps the greatest safeguard of all was that David was not, in fact, *agreeing to speak for money.* As he often said during the research for this book, he would have participated in this project even if there had been no financial incentive. He was telling his story in order to correct a published record of his life that had stood for over twenty-five years—a published record which expressly denied the extraordinary torments he had undergone and which, to David's everlasting horror, had led to similar anguish for untold numbers of children. Given the nature of this enterprise, no amount of money (I'm convinced) could have prompted David to lie about his past. And indeed, no one could have sat up with David until the small hours of the morning, night after night, and listened to him drag up memories of his blighted childhood, as I did, and doubt the veracity of his testimony.

Given my confidence that money played no part in tainting this story, I refrained from disclosing the details of my financial arrangement with David when writing the main body of this book. I do so now only to counter an insinuation made by John Money who, shortly before this book's publication, released a book of his own in which, at an effort at preemptive strike, he reprinted details of a gossip column that mentioned the size of the advance paid for this book and that moviemakers had become interested in David's story. "While money talks," he wrote, "it does not necessarily guarantee the truth." I do not think it is possible to read the final chapter of this book, in which David's long monologue is printed, and to feel that you are hearing money talking. Likewise, David's humiliating accounts of his junior high school years, when, in a bid to alleviate the unrelenting pressure of doctors and parents to have vaginal surgery, he actually attempted to behave as a girl— donning lipstick and skirts, attending school dances, allowing himself to be pecked on the cheek by a boy. Not until we began our deep interviews for the book did David dredge up this most shaming (but important) passage in his life. He had never mentioned it to Diamond and Sigmundson; he had refrained from mentioning it to me during the many months I interviewed him for *Rolling Stone*. That David should choose to volunteer this information to me for a book that he knew would be revealing his actual name, face, and location was my most convincing guarantee that, in participating with *As Nature Made Him*, David would allow nothing to stand in the way of the truth of his experience.

Of course, as we embarked on those interviews in late 1997, there was no predicting how the world would take David's story. It was one thing for him to have been written about in article-length stories and medical journals as "John/Joan," quite another for him to step out as David Reimer, in a book. Would he join the ignominious John Wayne Bobbitt as fodder for late-night talk show jokes? Would supermarket tabloid photographers camp out on his lawn to get photos of "the boy who was raised as a girl"? Thankfully, he was spared these indignities. Upon its publication in February 2000, his story was greeted with universal compassion and respect by readers. Letters and emails flooded in from people expressing their admiration for his courage and survival. His neighbors, friends, and coworkers at the slaughterhouse (which closed shortly before the book's publication) took the news of his past with equanimity. (Through a mutual friend, David was told that many of his coworkers had expressed sadness that David had never told them of his past.) Journalists and talk show hosts the world over requested interviews. David, standing behind his decision that his story should reach the widest possible audience, agreed to appear, undisguised, on a variety of these programs; among them, the *Oprah Winfrey Show*, *Dateline NBC*, and *Good Morning America* as well as a number of other TV and radio programs in the USA, Canada, Europe, and the Antipodes. In almost every instance, he was treated with remarkable sensitivity and tact by interviewers. David, in turn, refused to be just another entry in the unending parade of self-pitying victims who so often clutter our airwaves. Dry-eyed, forthright, blunt-spoken, he answered the questions put to him, never with an air of hoping to elicit pity (indeed, there is no emotion against which he responds with such impatience), and always with a finely calibrated sense of where the public's need to know ends and his own privacy begins. Asked by Oprah Winfrey about the phalloplasty which restored to him the ability to have sex with his wife, David said that it resembles a normal organ, then looked out over the audience and said: "And that's all I'm going to say about *that*"—which brought a round of cheers, laughter, and applause.

Once wholly anonymous, David is, today, often stopped on the street by strangers who recognize him and who wish to congratulate him for his strength. I happened to be with him in Manhattan after appearing live on *Good Morning America* when just such an encounter took place. A hurrying New Yorker emerged from the morning rush hour crowds on Fifth Avenue to seize David by the hand and tell him how he had inspired her. "You walk in the light, man!" she called out, as she moved back into the foot traffic. It was an extraordinary moment for both us. For over a year and a half, during our collaboration on the telling of David's story, I had listened to David discuss how his past had made him feel like a "freak"; I had listened to him describe how the history of lies that had surrounded his childhood had made it impossible for him to trust people; I had listened to him describe, with sometimes acid cynicism, his sense of the essential cruelty of humanity, perhaps the saddest legacy of his history of being ridiculed and rejected by his peers from kindergarten on. During those moments when that New Yorker held David's hand and poured out her heartfelt admiration for him, it was as if all those wounds were, for a moment, healed. And indeed, for several moments afterward, David was virtually speechless, simply smiling and saying, over and over, "How about that?"

Over the ensuing months, David would have many such encounters with strangers. "Some of them even ask for an autograph," he says, laughing. "I like it. For my whole life I felt like people are going to ridicule you if they learn the truth." Nor has the interest in David's story abated in the months since this book was published. Interview requests continue to come in, with regularity, from countries where foreign editions are now beginning to appear. Whenever possible, David tries to honor the requests for interviews.

"It's hard to talk about it all the time," he recently told me about the seemingly unending publicity blitz. "The memories flood back that much faster. And they're not good memories. But what choice do I have? No one else who's been through what I've been through seems to want to talk about it. I don't blame them. It's embarrassing. But if you're going to let people know the truth, you have no choice. It's the only way to change things."

Acknowledgments

=====

BESIDES THE REIMER family and all others named in this book who granted me interviews, I'd also like to acknowledge the crucial help of Mel Myers, Josh Weinstein, John Danakas, and Keith Black in Winnipeg; Dave Amber at the American Academy for the Advancement of Science in Washington, D.C.; Sara Pinto at the BBC in London; Miriam Zuger, whom I happened first to contact just days after the passing of her husband, Bernard, and who supplied me with reprints of his fascinating papers; Holly Devor, who has written two books on intersexuality; Edward Eichel who gave me the difficult-to-find *Paidiki* interview with John Money; Drs. Mariano and Marvin Tan who fielded endless e-mail queries about the twins' early lives; and photographer Ed Buryn who kindly sent me a copy of his book *Twin Births*. Thanks, also, to the staffs of the New York Academy of Medicine Library, the library of the New York Psychoanalytic Institute, and the

New York Society Library, where much of this book was written.

This book would not exist if not for my friend and longtime editor at *Rolling Stone*, Bob Love. He helped me shape and fine-tune the structure of the original article (which formed the narrative blueprint for *As Nature Made Him*), and he was always a patient sounding board for the ideas herein. Many thanks, too, to *Rolling Stone* editor and publisher Jann Wenner, who was passionate about this project from the outset, and whose reaction to the article's 17,500-word first draft was to bark, "It's great. Now gimme more!" Thanks also to the other people at *Rolling Stone* whose work on the article bears a lasting imprint on this book: Erika Fortgang, Tom Conroy, and Marian Berelowitz.

Closer to home, I'd like to thank certain members of my family for the grounding they gave me in medical and scientific terminology and ideas which made my journeying in these areas a good deal less disorienting than it would otherwise have been: my mother Carol, a registered nurse; my brother Ted, a neurosurgeon; and my late father, Vincent, who was for many years the chief of Urology at St. Michael's Hospital in Toronto and who, nightly, regaled me and my three siblings with tales from the medical world—including, in the early 1970s, the amazing news that when newborn boys lose their penis to circumcision they are turned into girls. Not himself a pediatric urologist, my father did not perform infant sex reassignments, but he (like the majority of medical men) accepted the psychological rationale behind them. I hope he would be proud of my efforts, with this book, to disseminate to the medical community (and world at large) contradictory evidence not available for the past three decades.

Many thanks to my agent, Lisa Bankoff, who made sure my proposal came before the eyes of the superb Robert Jones at HarperCollins. Not only did Robert give this book the most meticulous and artful edit, purging it of *longueurs*, repetition, and other maladies, he also somehow found the time to write explanations for each suggested change in the margin. I took them all. Thanks, too, to Fiona Hallowell at HarperCollins. Any errors of fact or interpretation, meanwhile, are my own.

I want to thank my wife, Donna Mehalko, who is the first person to read everything I write and upon whose instincts I rely utterly. Thanks, too, to my son John Vincent. Born eleven months into the process of my writing this book, he gave me, with his beloved presence, a special insight into the unimaginable horror faced by Ron and Janet Reimer all those years ago, and whose newborn crying, at times a distraction, was also a happy goad to keep at the computer and press on to the end.